Amish Vinegar Secrets

By Emily Thacker

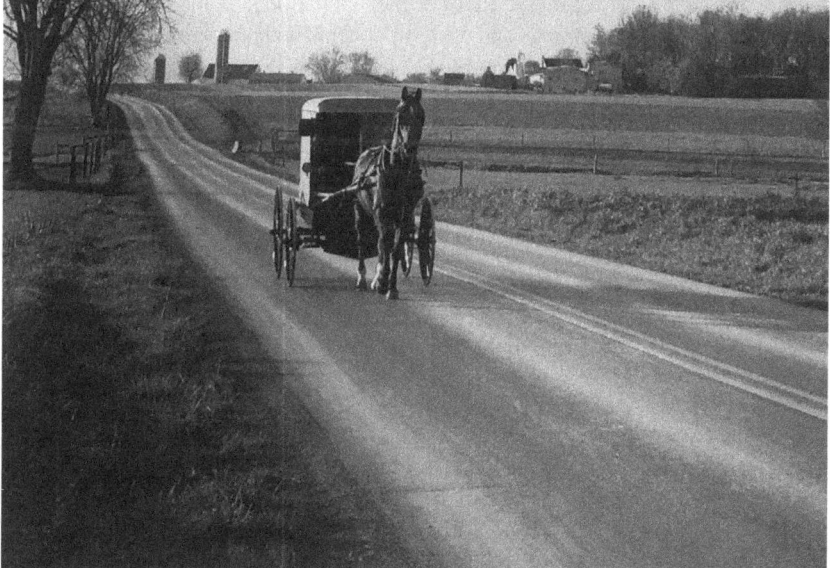

Published by:

James Direct Inc

500 S. Prospect Ave.

Hartville, Ohio 44632

U.S.A.

ISBN: 978-1-62397-076-5

Printing 12 11 10 9 8 7 6 5 4 3 2 1

First Edition   Copyright 2018   James Direct Inc

Table of Contents

Introduction

Welcome to the latest edition in my health series of natural home remedy books. It is with this book that I am probably most excited. After sharing nearly 30 years of research into the natural and holistic side of healing, I decided to take an entirely different approach to my exploration. Instead of looking ahead to what science has to offer next, I decided to look behind. And what I found was so obvious and so significant, I could not wait to share it with you.

When one thinks of a wholesome, simplified life brimming with nature and holistic health, one needs to look no further than Amish living. These quiet communities of plain people exemplify natural living.

While first thoughts of the Amish bring to mind images of quietly settled families amid abundant farmland, or even simple, buttonless clothing and old-fashioned values, a deeper look reveals surprising medical findings that have gone mostly unnoticed. It is easy to write off their use of homeopathic medicines and rudimentary lifestyle as antiquated, but scientific research reveals the Amish may have had it right all along.

Studies show that many chronic medical conditions we struggle with as a society simply do not exist, or occur to a much lesser degree, in Amish circles. For example, instances of asthma are found to be much less common in Amish children than those of the general population, even though Amish families are born and raised in farmland surrounded by hay and livestock – known catalysts for asthmatic attacks.

Amish communities also show less occurrences of certain types of cancer, including skin cancer, despite spending long days working under the blazing afternoon sun.

Heavy, calorie-laden meals that are rich in both fat and carbohydrates always seem to be associated with Amish mealtimes. Yet as a populace, they experience lower rates of cardiovascular disease than that of everyday society.

So, what can we attribute this to?

After delving further into the seemingly mysterious culture of the Amish, I discovered something not so mysterious. Their secret? Getting back to the basics of simple living may hold the answer to a long, healthy life. And, it could be just that easy.

What does basic, simple living entail? It means getting back to the basics consisting of a healthy, more natural diet, potent and effective home remedies based in natural substances, and a world free from toxic chemicals that, over time, can destroy the body's own natural defenses, possibly leaving it more susceptible to disease than ever before.

The Amish seem to take pride (for lack of a better term) in building up the body's immune system and preventing illness from taking hold. Modern medicine treats the symptoms of disease after sickness has already taken a stronghold. Amish medicine works the opposite way — preventing illness from occurring in the first place.

When sickness does occur, they treat it quickly and aggressively by natural means that do not simply mask symptoms, but work in conjunction with the body's own immune system to fight disease.

Even mundane cleaning comes down to choosing wholesome, natural cleaning options over today's commercial chemical-based cleaning solutions which oftentimes do more harm than good. Modern commercial cleaning products are full of toxic chemicals which can leave behind harmful residue long after cleaning has taken place. And oftentimes the very chemicals used to combat germs can actually build up a long term resistance in that bacteria, making it difficult, if not impossible, to truly eliminate.

So, what is the answer? A common thread through so much of natural healing and wholesome living can be found in one simple ingredient found in all Amish households – vinegar! It seems the Amish may have known all along the answers we have been searching so hard for.

Vinegar can be found not only in the pantries of Amish households, but also sold in their stores and used abundantly on their farms. It is a substance chock-full of nutrients, vitamins and minerals essential for good health. It can kill germs on contact, making vinegar an ideal cleaning solution, safe for both people and pets. And, it has a distinctive, robust flavor making it easy to incorporate into daily meals as a preventative medicine.

While modern science is working hard to reinvent the proverbial wheel, the Amish have long kept with the simple solutions that have worked best from the beginning.

This new book, *Amish Vinegar Secrets,* looks at ways to incorporate vinegar into everyday living for a better, healthier life. I am hopeful that you will gain something beneficial, and the information you find here to make a healthier, happier you!

All my best,

Emily Thacker

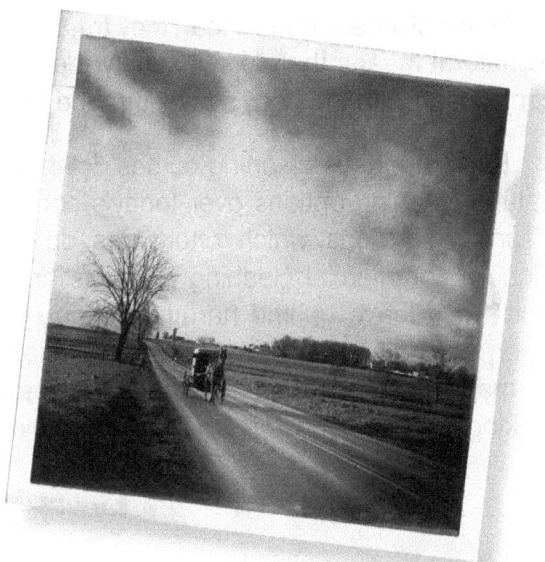

Chapter One

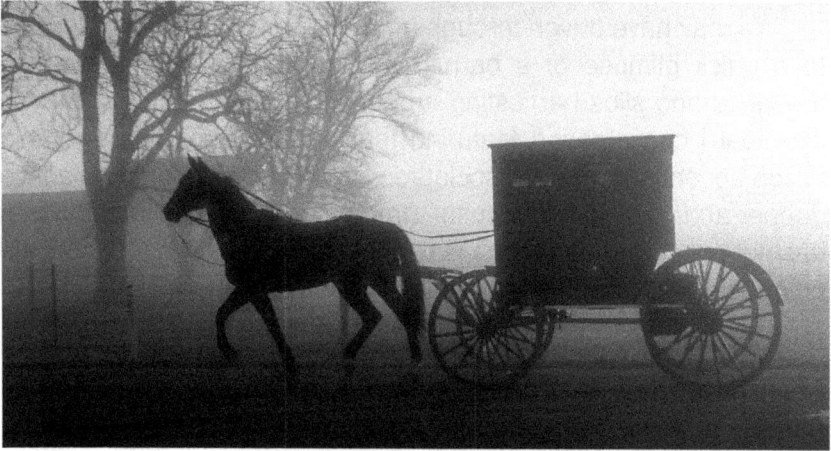

Why the Amish?

Most of us are familiar with the Amish name. One mention of it brings to mind images of plain clothes, horses and buggies, and abundant farmlands. They believe deeply in family and God, and encourage hard work – all the while eschewing modern technologies and everyday conveniences. The Amish are known for their modest and primitive way of life.

A leisurely stroll through Amish country brings sights, sounds and smells of a culture long past: no hurried lifestyle, just a reserved quietness. It is a culture steeped in tradition and rich in heritage. Their way of life is synonymous with simplicity, entrenched with firm family values and ethics.

The Amish live in close-knit communities that have chosen to separate themselves from the modern world. It is a culture void of electricity, automobiles and telephones. Yet even without these modern "necessities," the Amish are a people that thrive. Their barns and storehouses are always full, and their fields produce a rich harvest of crops.

We may have driven through an Amish village and were treated to a quick glimpse of a barn raising, watched children working the fields and silos harvesting a bountiful summer crop, or maybe overheard conversation featuring that distinct, thick Pennsylvania Dutch accent so widely associated with this group. But, look a little deeper and you will find a culture immersed in holistic tradition that has not only brought about a way of life based in strength and well-being, but also one of beauty, vitality and even longevity.

While most Amish sects will make use of institutional medicine when necessary, they much prefer natural healing remedies and a more traditional approach to a healthy lifestyle. They may live a quiet, understated life, but evidence of the reward of this natural lifestyle is easily observed.

Amish living is a sharp contrast to our busy, complicated lives, and a poignant reminder of more simple times long past. Times when we were not so hurried and families cherished moments of togetherness.

Somehow, modern living, and all its promises of convenience, has done little to foster more of those times. Many of today's technological advances, the very advances the Amish avoid, have fallen short of their promise of easing the daily workload and providing more discretionary time. Our lives are as busy as ever, with more time constraints and greater responsibility than ever before. Instead of leaving us with more time to spend at the family dinner table, microwaves have given us three minute meals (hardly nutritious) to consume in front of the evening television in a hurried rush.

The same can be said for some medical advances. While modern medicine has been truly miraculous and saved more lives than at any time in human history, it also comes with a calculated price. There is a corporate edge that has enabled some to become dependent on addictive medication, pay exuberant costs for that medication, and take risks with unintended side effects or harmful drug interactions.

So how is it that the Amish, living apart from modern society and all its technological advances, fare so well? Why do so many in their rural communities avoid the common ailments that seem to plague the rest of the general population? And what is the mind set of this fascinating culture that allows it to thrive while not participating with mainstream America? The answers to these questions help us better understand the Amish's natural approach to living.

Consider the flawless skin and rosy cheeks of Amish women. These women are known to have lower rates of skin cancer, even though they spend much of their days working outside in direct sunlight. Amish communities are filled with children working in silos and hay-filled barns packed with all types of livestock, yet their rate of being afflicted with asthma and allergies is less than that of other children their age. Men consume heavy, oftentimes fatty, meals and calorie-rich desserts, but are less afflicted with heart disease than the average American.

Research has shown that some of this can be attributed to genetics, and some to environmental circumstances. But, we have also learned that the Amish approach to a holistic style of living plays a very important role, as well.

The Amish perspective on health and wellness differs greatly from that of traditional medicine. Traditional medicine focuses on sickness-oriented solutions; it responds to the symptoms of an ailment after the fact. But, the Amish know the secret to healthy living begins by preventing disease *before* sickness sets in. And they accomplish this through a life replete of primal living.

The knowledge the Amish have held for generations, leaves science racing to catch up: The best way to "treat" a disease is to prevent it before it begins.

Natural healing and "folk medicine" play an integral part of Amish health, many remedies having been passed down for generations. They tend to rely heavily on medicinal herbs, poultices, salves, liniments, heat treatments and ointments.

Chiropractors and massotherapists are also used to treat headaches, back pain and muscle aches. In fact, some say that the Amish community is more accepting of holistic and natural healing practices than the country at large. One possible reason for the wide acceptance in Amish circles may be that natural medicine and healing remedies tend to be less invasive and not as expensive when compared to their more traditional counterparts.

Another factor that may influence the tendency toward natural home remedies over modern medicine is the avoidance of the use of pharmaceuticals. The standing thought being: why take a pill if a home healing remedy made with all-natural ingredients from the very farm you own can help ease my condition?

Amish health basically consists of a two-pronged approach: prevent illness before it strikes through healthy living, and treat unavoidable sicknesses and conditions using natural means whenever possible. Simple, but effective.

Preventative Health

These Plain people believe in preventative medicine by living a healthy, nature-based life. Illicit drug use is strictly prohibited, and in many sects, alcohol and tobacco. The concept of whole foods (food in its most natural state, void of chemicals and artificial additives) along with daily exercise is an innate part of life.

Their diet consists of fresh fruits and vegetables, homemade breads, and a variety of meats, dairy products and legumes. If you look closely at the meals they prepare, they are not necessarily low in calories. In fact, by most standards, the Amish diet would be considered "fattening." Yet, rates of obesity are again lower than the population at large (more about this in a later chapter), and we also see lower instances of diabetes and heart disease.

The Amish have immersed themselves in a healthy living cycle since childhood. They are proactive in establishing and maintaining their bodies for better health. As a whole, the Amish seem to have great success in preventing many sicknesses and diseases, in addition to staving off many life-threatening conditions.

And this way of thinking seems to be working.

Statistically, scientific research shows the Amish have lower rates of disease, such as diabetes, cardiovascular disease and even some cancers. A widely circulated article in the prestigious, *New England Journal of Medicine*, again details lower rates of asthma in Amish children compared with children in the general population. It is also believed that many in the Amish community may have stronger overall immune systems, helping to stave off disease.

Natural Healing
No matter how healthy a lifestyle one lives, sickness can still manage to find its way through. Even the Amish are not immune. And when disease does take hold, the Amish are some of the best practitioners of natural healing remedies. They are renowned for their deep knowledge of potent home remedies literally passed down from family to family. Simple, but effective remedies made from all-natural ingredients that work in conjunction with your body's own chemistry to boost the immune system and bring relief quickly and effectively.

And while many of their healing remedies also get a boost from additional common household herbs, the basis for much of their secret home remedies lies in common, everyday apple cider vinegar. Whether taken as a daily tonic to build the body strong and prevent future illness, or as a natural healing home remedy for various conditions, apple cider vinegar is the go-to for better health!

Apple cider vinegar can not only be used as a daily health tonic, but, the Amish also use vinegar liberally as a household cleaner, killing germs and further preventing the spread of illness and disease. It is considered a staple food in Amish households and readily available for an endless variety of uses.

In the chapters ahead, you will learn the secret of how the Amish incorporate vinegar in every facet of daily living to promote better health, wellness and vitality.

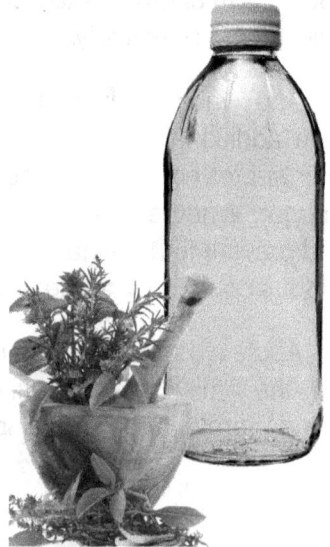

Chapter Two

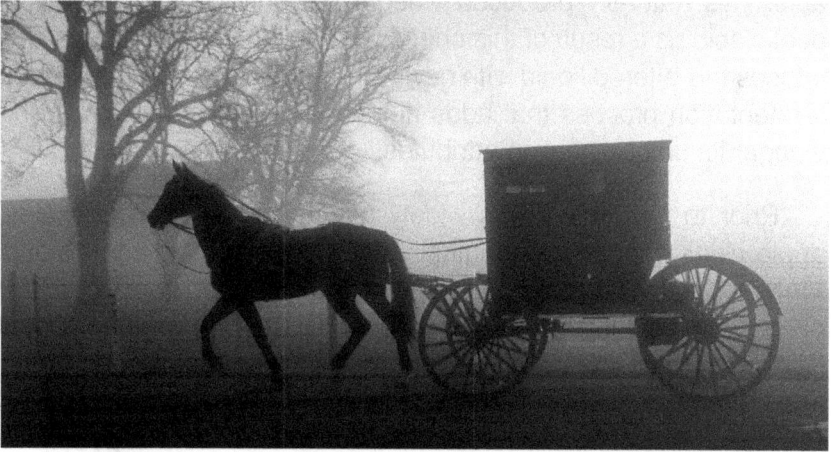

What is Apple Cider Vinegar?

What is apple cider vinegar, and why do the Amish use it so often in healing remedies?

Vinegar, by definition, is a liquid made up of water and acetic acid. The acetic acid in vinegar is formed during the fermentation process of ethanol. It is a complex substance containing additional trace elements, an assortment of healthy nutrients, enzymes and even flavorings.

Vinegar is one of the oldest and most versatile compositions on the planet. The English word "vinegar" is derived from the French "vinaigre" – "vin" meaning wine and "aigre" meaning sour. Translated literally, vinegar means "wine that has soured."

From a more technical standpoint, vinegar is the result of the oxidation-fermentation process of ethanol. Ethanol (ethyl alcohol) is then converted into acetic acid (vinegar) through an acetobacter, a living substance that oxidizes the alcohol, leaving behind acetic acid. The end result is a potent liquid containing 4% to 8% acetic acid. This naturally produced vinegar not only contains plenty of acetic acid as a result of this chemical reaction, but the action itself infuses this altered liquid with newly created enzymes. It is this very fermentation process that adds nutritional value and flavor, giving vinegar its unique healing attributes.

Prior to the time it was widely recognized in medical circles, apple cider vinegar was originally used to keep food from rotting. Vinegar's acidity inhibits bacterial growth, making it ideal for the preservation of food. It was poured over meats, fish, vegetables and fruits. Oftentimes the end result of fermentation tastes even better and more flavorful than the original food itself (for example, pickles). But soon, this bacterial inhibitor was found to be extremely useful in medical settings.

The Leap from Preservative to Healer
It is doubtful early users of vinegar were even aware of its chemical composition and the potent heath properties vinegar contained. Early on, vinegar was used as a crucial food preservative. Food that was submerged in vinegar retained both its color and flavor long after it should have spoiled. Soon, it was discovered that open, festering sores began to heal when doused with vinegar. Cooks in the kitchens of kings and doctors tending to the sick began to realize vinegar's unique and potent healing potential.

Eventually, vinegar's bacteria-inhibiting trait was used to treat a variety of common maladies such as sore throats, sprained and strained muscles, itchy skin, digestive issues and more. As the knowledge and understanding of vinegar's medicinal properties and potency grew, so did its uses, establishing itself as the hallmark treatment for hundreds of conditions and illnesses in the world of natural health remedies.

Making Vinegar Today
Science considers vinegar a complicated substance, overflowing with numerous flavors and aromas, immersed with a

wide assortment of enzymes, nutrients and trace elements. Fusion between the sweet, wooden storage barrels vinegar is aged in and the sharp sour zing of acetic acid, creates the best, most robust tasting vinegar.

Any plant that manufactures enough sugar to ferment into alcohol can be a parent to this substance. In addition to the obvious choice of apples, this includes pears, grapes, rice and even pineapple. Its distinctive flavor, aroma and healthfulness is derived from the elements found in the original food from which it was made. In addition, these unique characteristics leave a pleasant aroma and flavor directly reflecting its original food source.

Wine vinegar, like wine, can begin with either red or white grapes. Red wine vinegar is flavorful and intense, whereas white is apt to be a bit more astringent. Before processing the standardization of its acid content, wine vinegar has a higher natural concentration of acetic acid than apple cider vinegar. This is because grapes have a higher sugar content than apples.

Italy's famous **balsamic vinegar** is a specially aged wine vinegar. It is very dark, strongly aromatic and sweet. This is considered to be the very best, most concentrated vinegar. Sherry vinegar is a brownish amber color and has the woodsy, nutty taste and fragrance of Spanish sherry. It is not as sweet tasting as apple cider vinegar.

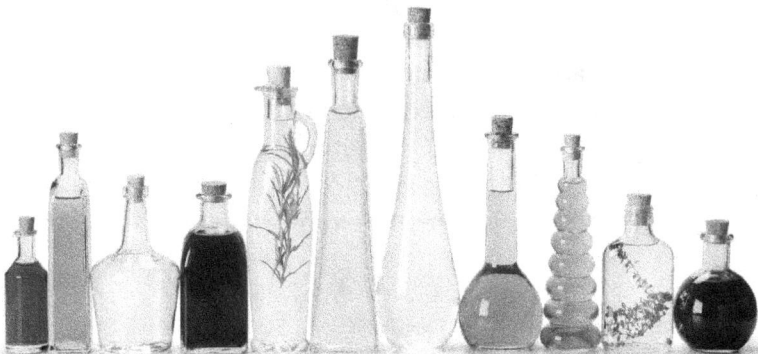

Sherry vinegar is a brownish amber color and has the woodsy, nutty taste and fragrance of Spanish sherry. It is not as sweet-tasting as apple cider vinegar.

Champagne vinegar is made from grapes picked before they are fully ripe. This vinegar is mild and delicate, which makes it a good choice as a base for flower-scented vinegars.

Malt vinegar begins with barley, which is then soaked in water, allowed to germinate and ultimately fermented into this dark English favorite. It is a robust, full-flavored vinegar and an essential ingredient of Worcestershire sauce.

Rice vinegar, at its best, most nutritious, is made from whole rice. Cost-conscious producers sometimes make lower grades from the lees left after the manufacture of rice wine. Rice vinegar is one of the mildest types and can be clear, red or dark brown in color. It is an integral part of both oriental cooking and Traditional Chinese Medicine (TCM).

Organic vinegar indicates a product that is produced without the use of chemical additives, from food which has been grown without the use of pesticides. And, good organic vinegar contains obvious remnants of the healthful food from which it was made. It should be a product that has not had its goodness filtered out, and not been over heated or over processed. Because organic vinegar can sometimes contain beneficial sediment at the bottom of the bottle, it may not be as 'pretty' as pasteurized, super-filtered varieties.

Yeast is the key converter in the vinegar-making process, as its acetobacters cause the alcohol to change into acetic acid. Most historians agree that vinegar probably began as a wine that was exposed to oxygen in the air we breathe. Yeasts that were found naturally in wine helped ferment it into what we today refer to as vinegar.

Simply put, vinegar is formed when a sugary liquid, such as you would find in pureed apples, is changed into an alcoholic solution through a yeast reaction or by fermentation. Then, this chemical reaction is changed yet again, ending in an acetic acid containing solution.

While this describes the technical aspect of vinegar, it is really so much more!

Apple Cider Vinegar versus White Vinegar

Some of the most common questions asked when discussing vinegar pertains to the difference between apple cider vinegar and white vinegar.

"What is the difference between the two?"

"Which type of vinegar is best for home remedies?"

"Can I use white vinegar for cleaning?"

While both are true vinegars, apple cider vinegar and white vinegar are two very different types, each with their own unique makeup, benefits and effective uses.

Apple cider vinegar is made from a wide variety of whole apples that have been chopped, ground or pureed into smaller pieces. Sometimes, the apples' peeling and cores are also used in this kind of vinegar. Depending upon which variety of apple is used, sweet, tart and even crab apples can help add flavor and aroma to apple cider vinegar's taste. Each apple brings its own unique taste and attributes to the final product.

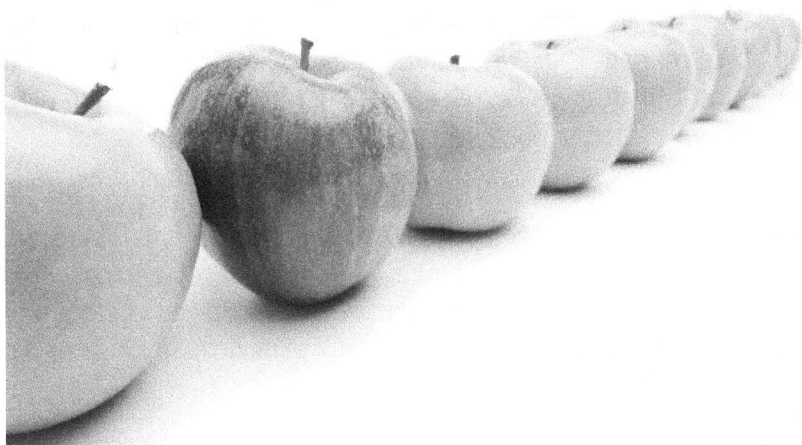

Cut apples are permitted to "breathe" for a period of time, allowing tannins to form as the apples react with air. This process gives apple cider vinegar its rich flavor and color. Juice is then pressed or squeezed from the apples through a special press, and then permitted to ferment into a hard cider. These fermented apples give apple cider vinegar the aroma it is noted for. As the hard cider ferments even longer, vinegar is formed.

Apple cider vinegar is a healthy, robust vinegar with a wide range of uses. It is an excellent choice for most pickling needs, cooking purposes, and skin and hair treatments. It has a taste much like rice vinegar and can be used interchangeably in recipes. Apple cider vinegar contains a healthy dose of pectin. This water-soluble fiber is easily dissolved in the body's digestive system, but remains in the body longer than insoluble fibers. Apple cider vinegar is notably packed with a storehouse of vitamins and minerals which are of enormous benefit to the human body. These nutrients can help restore depleted elements within the body or bring numerous health benefits to those suffering from an array of ailments and conditions.

White vinegar, also called distilled vinegar, is derived from corn which is distilled into corn alcohol. Additional ingredients are added to the corn alcohol and allowed to ferment, forming white vinegar. This fermentation process is complete once all of the alcohol has left the product, leaving only white vinegar behind. Just like its cousin, apple cider vinegar, white vinegar is completely natural.

White vinegar can also be made from leftover food by-products. These by-products tend to be not only plentiful, but inexpensive. This is the reason white vinegar lacks the sweet, distinctive aroma associated with fruit-based vinegars, such as the more common apple cider vinegar.

While white vinegar can still be a good choice for the pickling and preservation of foods, it does lack the rich color that apple cider vinegar boasts. This makes white vinegar a better choice when used on light-colored vegetables, such as cauliflower, potatoes or foods like white onions. It also injects less of its own flavor, so there is less interference with the flavoring of certain delicate herbs.

Because white vinegar is manufactured from corn, it is considered one of the least expensive vinegars on the market. This means white vinegar is a superb choice for most cleaning projects, as its cheaper price allows for more liberal usage, all while keeping the same potency as other more costly vinegars. White vinegar's lack of color can also make it a good choice for some cleaning projects, as it does not stain delicate cloths and materials.

Apple Cider Vinegar for Better Health
Apple cider vinegar is a natural healing solution. It contains unique medicinal properties that are not only potent, but highly effective in preventing and eliminating illness. It also promotes health and healing to already infected and ailing tissue, killing bacteria while still protecting delicate skin areas.

Scientific research indicates that apple cider vinegar is rich in numerous vitamins and minerals the human body craves for proper function. Apple cider vinegar is fat free, and contains less than 30 calories and only 2 milligrams of sodium in an *entire cup,* making it an outstanding health choice for those watching caloric or sodium intake.

Science has discovered more than 90 different compounds or components in vinegar, most of which have tremendous health benefits to the human body. These substances include:

- 33 carbonyls
- 13 phenols
- 7 bases
- 4 acids

- 11 alcohols
- 8 esters
- 7 hydrocarbons
- 3 furans

At one time, many researchers believed white vinegar did not contain the beneficial attributes that its close cousin possesses. But further testing and research revealed that white vinegar does contain a storehouse of essential nutrients. While apple cider vinegar still boasts a more potent health brew of these substances, white vinegar is now also revered as a health remedy in its own right.

A few of these essential health substances which can be found in white or distilled vinegar include:

- Protein
- Phosphorus
- Potassium
- Carbohydrates
- Vitamin D
- Zinc
- Magnesium
- Riboflavin (vitamin B-2)
- Calcium
- Iron
- Fiber
- Vitamin A
- Folacin
- Niacin
- Thiamin (vitamin B-1)
- Ascorbic acid (vitamin C)

While researchers are excited about the possible healing potential of these newly found health substances in white vinegar, apple cider vinegar's list of essential qualities is unparalleled. Apple cider vinegar exhibits an even more impressive list of healing compositions, such as:

- Calcium
- Iron
- Vitamin A
- Zinc
- Magnesium
- Riboflavin (vitamin B-2)
- Vitamin B-6
- Copper
- Manganese
- Isoleucine
- Leucine
- Methionine
- Tyrosine
- Arginine
- Histidine
- Aspartic acid
- Glycine
- Serine
- Phosphorus
- Potassium
- Folate
- Niacin
- Thiamin (vitamin B-1)
- Ascorbic acid (vitamin C)
- Pantothenic acid
- Potassium
- Tryptophan
- Threonine
- Lysine
- Cystine
- Valine
- Phenylalanine
- Alanine
- Glutamic acid
- Proline

Because different vinegars, such as balsamic, wine, rice and champagne vinegars are derived from other sources before fermentation, each brings its own chemical composition and qualities to the table. While these different sources can sometimes confuse scientists on why vinegar is such as amazing healing agent, they do agree that vinegar itself contains some very unusual properties that make it conducive to healing and healthier lifestyles.

Physicians know that the human body depends on very tiny amounts of hundreds as of yet largely unidentified compounds. Scientific research in the field of nutrition are constantly discovering new enzymes, amino acids and other substances essential to the body for complete health. Exactly how the human body uses many of these elements still eludes science. But, doctors do know that even a tiny deficiency of an essential health element can result in sickness, premature aging or damage to healthy brain tissue. The best advice today's scientists can give us to this point, is to eat a wide assortment of fresh foods, giving the body a wide spectrum of necessary nutrients.

So, what happens when the body becomes depleted of these essential nutrients? Sickness, disease and a multitude of conditions can follow. Some believe vinegar may be as close as we will ever come to a universal remedy for these depleted nutrients. It also comes with a host of health-related attributes that are still being sorted out and catalogued. Many of these qualities can be game changers for someone who is dealing with health issues or wishes to prevent certain health problems altogether.

Can the Compounds in Apple Cider Vinegar Really Make a Difference Toward Better Health?

So how do these attributes actually work, and why are they important? This list of tiny nutrients, minerals and other health substances all work together forming themselves into much larger, more potent traits essential to health and healing. Take a look at this list of vinegar qualities and what each has to offer the human body. It is a pretty impressive list of healing properties that one would be hard pressed to find in another single natural health substance:

Antiseptic
Infection preventer and disease fighter; prohibits the growth and spread of infections. Works to prevent the growth of illness-causing microorganisms in the body.

Antibiotic
Used in the prevention or fight of infectious disease; weakens and kills certain types of harmful bacteria and fungus.

Antibacterial
Kills bacteria and inhibits the spread or growth of bacteria.

Anti-inflammatory
Helps to inhibit or prevent swelling and inflammation throughout the human body in joints, muscles and other areas.

Antifungal
Destroys or weakens harmful viruses; can also inhibit the spread of a virus and stop its growth.

Antioxidant
Works to inhibit oxidation within the human body. Antioxidants protect delicate cells within the body from dangerous free radicals known to promote many types of cancers.

Antimicrobial
Works to inhibit the spread and potency of microorganisms, and depending on the microorganism itself, kill some altogether.

All of these characteristics work together to not only promote better health and healing, but in many cases prevent illness from occurring in the first place. Whether using vinegar as an oral tonic, antiseptic medicinal emulsion, or to clean away germs and bacteria from your home, vinegar is an exceptional natural health solution.

Vinegar and Fiber
Vinegar contains an arsenal of complex carbohydrates, as well as a good dose of dietary fiber. Both complex carbohydrates and

dietary fiber have been recommended by the U.S. Surgeon General to help build resistance to cancer.

There are different types of fiber. Some are water soluble and some not. A water-soluble fiber soaks up water (adding bulk), but also has the power to interact with the body. Insoluble fibers soak up water (adding bulk), but do not interact with the body in the same complex manner soluble fibers do.

When vinegar is made from fresh, natural apples it contains a healthy dose of pectin. Pectin is considered a soluble fiber. It dissolves in water, making it very available for the body to use. In addition to soaking up water, it slows down the absorption of food and liquid in the intestines. Therefore, it remains in the body longer than an insoluble fiber.

An insoluble fiber, such as wheat bran, rushes through the system. Particularly, it rushes through the intestines, giving it laxative properties. Fibers such as wheat bran also produce large amounts of gas.

As pectin, the fiber found in apple cider vinegar, works its slow, gentle way through the digestive system, it binds to cholesterol. Pectin then pulls the bound cholesterol out of the body, reducing its footprint in the system. Less cholesterol in the body makes for a reduced risk of cardiovascular problems, such as heart attacks and strokes.

Vinegar and Digestion
Apple cider vinegar is very similar to the chemicals found naturally in the stomach. Because of this, it has traditionally been hailed as an aid to digestion. And in improving digestion, it can improve the overall metabolism of the body.

Vinegar is also considered by many to be able to attack and kill harmful bacteria which has invaded the body's digestive tract. This may lessen the likelihood of the body developing toxemia and other blood-borne infections.

Vinegar, Beta Carotene and Cancer

Aging, heart disease, cancer and cataracts are symptoms of the harm done to the human body by free radicals, the "loose cannons" of the cell world. They damage chromosomes and are believed to be responsible for many of the physical changes associated with aging.

Free radicals roam through nature in the form of plants, animals and humans, bouncing from cell to cell, damaging each in turn. Antioxidants absorb these free radicals, rendering them harmless. Beta carotene, a carotenoid found in vinegar, is a powerful antioxidant.

Carotenoid occurs naturally in plants such as apples. Beta carotene found in vinegar is already in a natural, easy to digest form. One example of how this antioxidant contributes to maintaining good health is the way it protects the eye from cataracts. Cataract development is related to oxidation of the eye's lens. This happens when free radicals alter its structure. Studies show that eating healthy amounts of antioxidant-containing foods decreases the risk of forming cataracts.

A correlation between eating foods containing beta carotene and a lower risk of cancer has been documented, as well. Researchers, in more than 70 different studies, agree beta carotene lowers the risk of getting cancer. They include those at the State University of New York at Stony Brook, the University of Western Ontario in Canada, Tufts University and Johns Hopkins School of Medicine.

In addition to giving cancer protection, beta carotene boosts the body's own immune system. It works by attacking the free radicals which destroy the immune system itself.

Carotenoids are also the body's raw material for producing vitamin A, another potent antioxidant. They act together to protect from cancers associated with chemical toxins. According to National Cancer Research in England, when the body does not get enough vitamin A, it is particularly susceptible to cancers of the respiratory system, bladder and colon.

Vinegar and Memory

According to medical studies, the three most common causes of memory loss are Alzheimer's disease, multi-infarct dementia (multiple strokes) and alcohol abuse. Many older patients also endure mental impairment caused by poor nutrition and reactions to prescription medications. While these conditions were once thought to be just another unavoidable sign of aging, new science tells us different.

Too often memory loss in individuals who are over age 55 is treated as if it were irreversible or inevitable. Yet information continues to indicate that the cause of many memory loss issues can be successfully treated. More physicians are echoing the words of one specialist, "…several of the causes are treatable, resulting in an arrest or actual reversal of the symptoms."

Nutrition is an important consideration when evaluating risk factors for memory loss, and to reverse damage which has already occurred. A healthy diet can decrease the likelihood of stroke by lowering cholesterol. It can also protect the mind from some of the worse causes of loss of mental function. The *Journal of the American Dietetic Association* puts it this way:

"Some forms of dementia, those due to excessive alcohol intake or vitamin deficiency, may be entirely preventable and partially reversible through diet."

The journal goes on to say:

"In all types of dementia, adequate nutrition may improve physical well-being, help maximize the patients' functioning and improve the quality of life."

Some studies indicate nutritional deficiencies are a problem for 36% of the over 80-year-old population. And, nearly half of all nursing home patients have been shown to have at least some vitamin or mineral deficiency. These decreased levels of vitamins and minerals are important because they can contribute to loss of mental ability. For example, memory loss is more frequent in patients who have lower than normal blood levels of vitamin B-12 and folate.

Apple cider vinegar supplies a balanced dose of vital amino acids, vitamins and minerals that both the mind and body require for good health.

Vinegar and Blood Sugar

A number of studies show a possible link between the intake of apple cider vinegar and the management of the body's blood sugar levels. One promising study in particular indicates that lab rats receiving doses of apple cider vinegar showed lower levels of LDL and A1C.

And a research study out of Arizona State University found that participants taking apple cider vinegar diluted in water with an additive of saccharine were able to lower their blood sugar levels following meals.

While both of these studies are not definitive, they certainly show promise to those suffering from diabetes.

What Does the Science Say?

Enthusiasts of apple cider vinegar can recite a long list of conditions it is reported to be able to either prevent or cure. It is claimed that vinegar can do everything from aiding digestion, balancing pH levels in the skin, banishing arthritis, destroying infection and forestalling osteoporosis to controlling weight, preserving memory, protecting the brain from aging and even preventing some cancers. Medical research's most recent findings have much to say on this very subject, and much of it is extremely promising.

Ohio State University's hospital is currently prescribing vinegar irrigation treatment for chronic middle ear infections. At the same time, The American Academy of Otolaryngology also suggests using a mixture of vinegar and alcohol to prevent swimmer's ear infections.

Doctors are currently considering treating some eye infections with diluted vinegar. Right now, they are using it as a hospital disinfectant. One example of this use can be found at Yale-New Haven Hospital. When post-surgery eye infections became a problem, their Department of Bacteriology solved the issue with common vinegar. The hospital began routinely cleaning the scrub-room sink with a 1/2% solution of ordinary household vinegar. It worked better at eliminating bacteria than the commercial product it replaced.

Reports out of Western Michigan University indicate vinegar can be used to increase the accuracy of conventional tests for cervical cancer. This new, vinegar-based test allows physicians to check for cancer that may not have been detected by the more familiar Pap test alone.

A study by the *Journal of Diabetes Research* shows that vinegar reduces hypoglycemia in type 2 Diabetes patients.

Vinegar supplements have been added to patient diets at the A.P. John Institute for Cancer Research, believing that vinegar can help in "shutting off cancer cells energy and causing them to die off."

Research by Dr. Yoshio Takino of Shizuoka University in Japan proved vinegar helps to maintain a healthy body and slow aging by preventing the formation of two fatty peroxides. This action deals with both damaging free radicals and cholesterol formations that can build up on the walls of blood vessels.

We also know that consuming carotenoid rich vegetables and fruits can be a preventative against skin cancer.

Depression can sometimes be linked to a deficiency of folic acid, calcium, iron, copper, magnesium or potassium – all nutrients found in apple cider vinegar.

Confusion and memory loss can be caused by too little vitamin B-12 or folic acid.

Studies also show that breast and prostate cancers seem to be restrained by lycopene, also found in vinegar.

Research indicates arthritis inflammation has been reduced when thiamin, B-6 and B-12 were added to standard medical treatments, sometimes in as little time as one week.

Each of these deals with nutrients or minerals that are associated with apple cider vinegar.

Amish Have Been Using Vinegar for Generations

With Amish households already considering vinegar a kitchen pantry necessity and benefitting from generations of home remedy solutions, the Amish are at a distinct advantage health-wise. They possess a deep knowledge of a multitude of ways to use apple cider vinegar's health qualities to their advantage, and incorporate vinegar into their daily life in the form of tonics, remedies, and even general cooking for better health.

Simply put, the Amish can effortlessly enjoy the healing benefits of vinegar, since it is already such a cornerstone in their world. They liberally use vinegar in daily recipes, use it as the foundation of tonics and poultices to treat illness and injury, and wipe, spray and pour it to clean and disinfect, harnessing its every possible use! In fact, while we are just delving into the world of apple cider vinegar, it has already become the product-of-choice for Amish families and their healthy lifestyle.

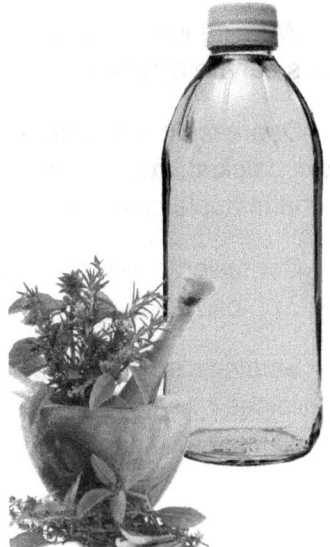

Chapter Three

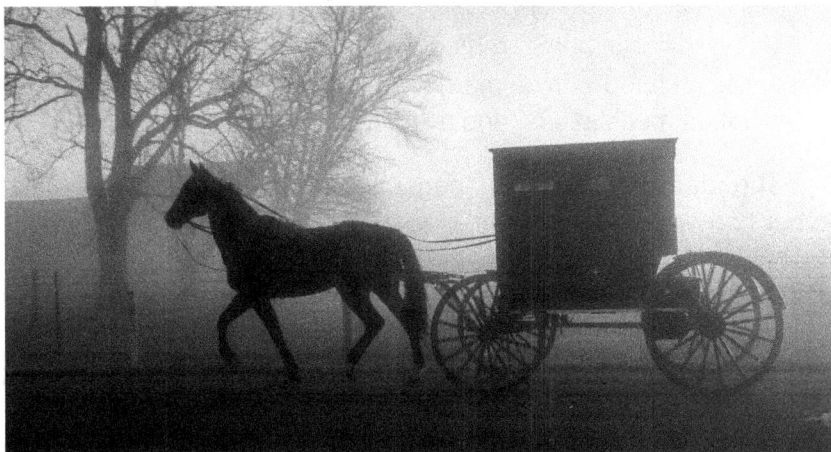

Amish Home Remedies

No one does natural healing and prevention better than the Amish! Tightly woven into their way of life are threads of self-reliance and natural living. To this effect, Amish folk have long used apple cider vinegar in all aspects of life, and can be found in virtually every Amish household. Apple cider vinegar is used as a way to maintain general good health, prevent sickness and disease, and control weight gain. It is a go-to remedy for everything from digestive ailments to coughs and colds, to asthma, allergies and breathing difficulties. Apple cider vinegar has even been used to relieve and control headaches, ease arthritis pain, and treat strains and sprains.

Best of all, science is finally catching up to what the Amish have known for generations:

- There are no harmful side-effects

- No dangerous drug interactions

- Vinegar is all natural
- It is packed with nutrients essential to healthy living

Using natural home remedies may help avoid harmful side effects associated with so many over-the-counter drug store pills or prescription medications, and avoid drug interactions.

The idea behind using vinegar as a home remedy, much like other homeopathic solutions, is to use the best qualities of vinegar to help strengthen the body's own undernourished or nutrient-depleted immune system to fight troublesome conditions. Vinegar can help reduce inflammation and swelling throughout the body, regulate pH levels, rid the body of harmful microorganisms, protect delicate cells from cancer-causing free radicals and even restore lost enzymes to the body that are vital for good health. Its antiseptic properties can work outside the body to kill harmful bacteria on cuts and scrapes, or ease the pain of muscle aches and sprains.

One of the greatest benefits to using apple cider vinegar as a home health remedy is promoting the growth of beneficial bacteria in the body to keep disease-producing germs in check. For example, human intestines contain millions of good bacteria, such as bifidus and lactobacillus, to keep the gastrointestinal tract healthy and disease free. Keeping "good" bacteria in the intestines also:

- Supports the immune system
- Helps digest food
- Manufactures some vitamins
- Keeps the intestines acidic
- Discourages illnesses caused by E. coli and clostridia bacteria

For the most part, apple cider vinegar tends to be the better choice for home remedies, due to the fact that it contains so many more vital nutrients and minerals, than its white vinegar counterpart. Remember that whatever the original food source the vinegar has been made from carries its health traits into the final vinegar product. So, apple-based apple cider vinegar, much like many of the fruit vinegars, would inherently contain more trace vitamins, minerals and nutrients than that of corn-based white vinegar.

Even though our lives tend to run at a faster pace than that of the Amish, there are Amish secrets we can incorporate into our daily routines for better health. Is vinegar a cure-all for everything that ails us? Probably not. And some remedies that began as folklore are still passed down from family to family. But others have shown great success in helping to alleviate infection and illness. It's up to you to determine how these will work for you and your family.

Historically, infections on the face, around the eyes and in the ears have been treated with a solution of vinegar and water. It works because vinegar is antiseptic (kills germs on contact) and antibiotic (contains bacteria which is unfriendly to infectious microorganisms).

More recently, vinegar has been used to treat chronic middle ear diseases when traditional drug-based methods fail. Remember, many of these remedies may require the benefit of time to begin working. While an upset stomach may be eased right away, relief from arthritis may require a couple of weeks to achieve. For instances like this, you may wish to try a topical treatment in conjunction with an oral tonic for immediate relief while you are waiting for the oral to take effect.

As with any new home remedy treatment, always consult a trusted healthcare provider prior to beginning, including the use of vinegar.

You will also notice that for some remedies, more than one remedy will be listed. The beauty of these entries is that they are ever changing from generation to generation. You may find that one is more palatable than another, or you may get an added health boost from an additional ingredient. Families have developed their own variations over time, as reflected in the wide variety of options listed here. Home remedies tend to be a very personal choice. Everybody responds differently to different treatments, so enjoy discovering which remedy might be best for you, your body and your personal situation, and make adjustments as needed.

So, let's get started.

The best way to fight disease is to curb it before it happens. Do you want an easy way to incorporate vinegar into your daily health routine? Try a little vinegar each day to keep the maladies away. Sometimes the best, most simple way to accomplish this is a quick teaspoon of apple cider vinegar first thing in the morning. Additional ideas follow.

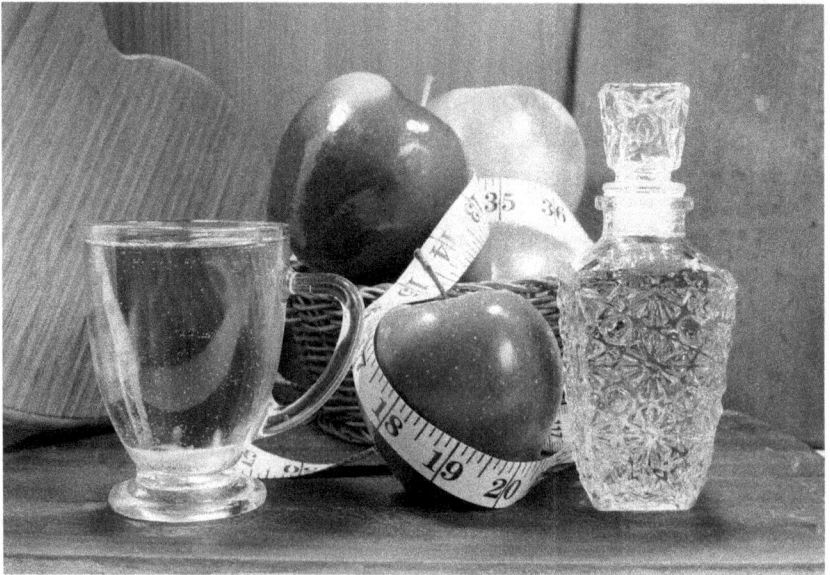

PREVENTATIVE VINEGAR REMEDIES

The "Original" Vinegar Tonic
1 tablespoon apple cider vinegar
8 ounce glass of water

Combine together and drink once a day.

Daily Vinegar Tonic #2
1 tablespoon apple cider vinegar
1 teaspoon honey
8 ounce glass of water

Combine both ingredients together and drink one to three times a day.

Daily Vinegar Tonic #3
2 tablespoons apple cider vinegar
1 teaspoon honey
8 ounce glass of water

Combine together and drink before dinner.

Daily Vinegar Serum
1 tablespoon apple cider vinegar
1 teaspoon honey

Combine and enjoy, with or without an 8 ounce glass of water.

Vinegar Detox
2 tablespoons apple cider vinegar
8 ounces warm water
1 tablespoons lemon juice
1 teaspoon honey (local, raw honey works best)
1/4 teaspoon ginger

Mix all ingredients together and drink while warm.

HOME REMEDIES

Acid Reflux
1 teaspoon apple cider vinegar
1 cup water

Mix apple cider vinegar into a glass of water and drink for instant relief of acid reflux.

Allergies (seasonal)
1 tablespoon apple cider vinegar
2 teaspoons honey
1 cup water

Combine vinegar and honey in a glass of water. Drink once in the morning and once in the evening to stave off seasonal allergies.

Arthritis
1 teaspoon apple cider vinegar
1 teaspoon honey
1 cup warm water

Combine vinegar and honey in a teacup or glass. Add warm water and stir until mixed, like a tea. Drink one glass in the morning, and a second glass before bedtime.

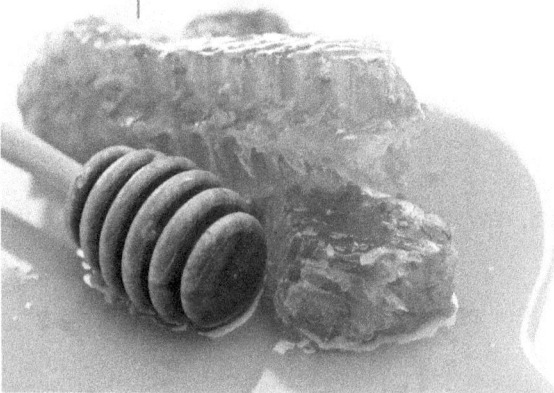

Arthritis
1 tablespoon apple cider vinegar
1/2 grapefruit
2 stalks celery
1 orange
1 lemon
4 cups water
1 tablespoon salt

Cut the celery, orange, grapefruit and lemon into chunks, leaving the peelings on the fruit. Simmer uncovered in water for one hour until ingredients are tender and soft. Press the softened ingredients through a jelly bag or tight sieve. Stir in vinegar and salt.

When ready to use, combine 1/4 cup of this mixture into a full glass of water. Drink one glass in the morning and a second glass in the evening.

Arthritis Tonic
2 teaspoons apple cider vinegar
1 cup water

Combine vinegar and water. Drink this combination before each meal, three times a day.

Arthritis
1 cup apple cider vinegar
1/2 cup honey
1/2 cup blueberries
1/2 cup raspberries
1 teaspoon lemon juice

Combine all ingredients in a blender. Take 2 to 3 tablespoons a day for pain relief.

Arthritis Poultice (DO NOT INGEST)
1/2 cup apple cider vinegar
2 egg whites
1/2 cup turpentine
1/4 cup olive oil

Combine all ingredients in a bowl or small disposable tub. Using a soft cloth, massage mixture into joints for relief from arthritis pain. Do NOT ingest. If desired, turpentine can be omitted from recipe.

Athlete's Foot
1 cup apple cider vinegar
5 cups water

Combine vinegar and water in a large bowl. Soak socks or nylons for 30 minutes before regular wash.

Asthma
Apple cider vinegar
Gauze pads
Rubber bands

Acupressure can be used to help alleviate the symptoms of asthma. Soak a gauze pad in vinegar, barely ridding the excess. Use the rubber bands to hold the gauze pads in place on the inside of the wrists. Be sure the rubber bands are tight enough to hold the pads in place, but not too tight to interrupt circulation or become uncomfortable.

Backaches
2 cups apple cider vinegar
warm bath water

Fill bath with warm water and add apple cider vinegar. Soak in tub for 20 minutes for relief from backaches.

Bladder Infection
1 tablespoon vinegar
1 cup water

Combine vinegar and water in a glass and drink 2 to 3 times a day to end bladder infection.

Bladder Infection
See also "Urinary Tract Infection"

Boils (poultice)
1 cup vinegar
1/4 cup fresh willow twigs, broken
clean, soft cloth

Simmer vinegar and fresh willow twigs on low heat until twigs are tender. Use liquid to coat a soft cloth and use as a poultice on tender skin boils.

Calluses
Apple cider vinegar
Slice stale bread
Tape

Dip half a slice of stale bread in apple cider vinegar, and secure in place on top of calluses before bed. Remove in the morning.

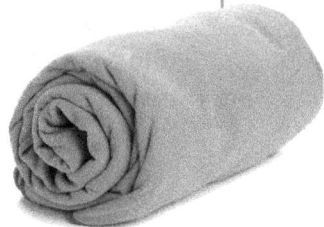

Cholesterol

The idea behind this remedy is knowing that pectin, found abundantly in all types of apples, slows the body's absorption of food in the intestines, giving it extra time to bind to cholesterol.

1 cup apple cider vinegar
2 cups chopped apples
1/2 cup honey
1/2 teaspoon nutmeg
1/2 teaspoon cinnamon

Place apples in a blender adding all other ingredients until well combined. Sip a few teaspoons of this fortified vinegar throughout the day.

Colds

apple cider vinegar
cayenne pepper
8" square of brown paper (grocery bag)

Soak an 8" square of brown paper in apple cider vinegar. Sprinkle one side of the wet brown paper with cayenne pepper and lay it directly on the chest for 15 to 20 minutes. Remove the used paper, and wash the chest clean, taking care not to become chilled.

Congestion

apple cider vinegar
soft, clean cloths

Soak soft, clean cloths in apple cider vinegar and wrap around wrists as bedtime to help ease congestion and breathe better at night.

Congestion
1/4 cup apple cider vinegar
vaporizer

Add apple cider vinegar to vaporizer water and allow vinegar vapors to penetrate the air. Breathing this will help ease congestion and allow for easier breathing.

Congestion
1 cup apple cider vinegar
1-2 tablespoons honey
1 clove garlic, mashed
pinch cayenne pepper

Mix all ingredients in a small bowl, and gently sip throughout the day to relief congestion.

Congestion
See also "Nasal Congestion"

Constipation
2 tablespoons apple cider vinegar
1 teaspoon lemon juice
1 cup water

Add vinegar and lemon juice to a glass of water, drinking 3 times a day to end constipation.

Constipation
2 tablespoons apple cider vinegar
1 cup apple juice

Add apple cider vinegar to a cup of apple juice and drink 2 to 3 times a day. The extra pectin in apple juice will work with the apple cider vinegar to end constipation.

Corns
See "Calluses"

Cough
1 cup apple cider vinegar
1-2 tablespoons honey
1 clove garlic, mashed

Combine all ingredients in a small bowl. Warm a small amount of solution and sip gently throughout the day to ease a nagging cough.

Cough
apple cider vinegar, undiluted

Sprinkle a clean pillowcase with apple cider vinegar before bedtime to soothe a dry night cough.

Diabetes
2 tablespoons apple cider vinegar
1 cup water

Combine apple cider vinegar and water and drink a few minutes before a meal to help stabilize blood sugar levels.

Diabetes
2 tablespoons apple cider vinegar
1/8 teaspoon salt
1 cup water

Combine all ingredients in a drinking glass and enjoy twice a day. This solution should be avoided by people who need to watch their sodium intake, since extra salt is added.

Diarrhea
1 teaspoon vinegar
1 cup water

Mix apple cider vinegar in a glass of water and drink 2 to 4 times a day to eliminate diarrhea.

Diarrhea
2 tablespoons apple cider vinegar
1 teaspoon honey
1 cup water

Combine vinegar and honey in a glass of water. Drink 3 to 4 times a day until diarrhea subsides. Will not only ease diarrhea, but will also help avoid dehydration common with diarrhea.

Digestion Problems
See "Stomach" issues
See "Food Poisoning Prevention"

Ear Infection
1 teaspoon apple cider vinegar

Tilt head toward the shoulder with ear facing the ceiling. Pour a teaspoonful of vinegar into the ear canal, making sure solution flows all the way down to the infection. Keep vinegar in ear for 30 seconds, and then tip ear upright to drain vinegar on a paper towel. Repeat three times a day until ear infection has cleared.

A straw can also be used to easily drop vinegar into the ear canal. Just be sure NOT to place the straw itself into the ear.

Ear Infection Prevention

Great solution to use after swimming in a pond or lake to prevent water-borne infections from settling in the ear.

3 tablespoons distilled vinegar
3 tablespoons rubbing alcohol

Combine both ingredients together and, using an eye dropper, gently rinse ear canal to eliminate any bacteria.

Eczema

2 teaspoons apple cider vinegar
1 teaspoon honey
1 cup water

Add vinegar and honey to glass of water. Consume mixture 2 to 3 times a day, for one week.

Eczema

apple cider vinegar
soft cloth

Soak a soft, clean cloth with undiluted apple cider vinegar and use to gently dab onto areas of skin effected with eczema.

Electrolytes

1 tablespoon apple cider vinegar
1 cup water

Mix a tablespoon of apple cider vinegar into a glass of water to restore depleted electrolytes after work-outs or long days working in the hot sun. This is also an excellent remedy to restore essential electrolytes when dehydrated due to illness.

Fatigue

1 teaspoon apple cider vinegar
1 teaspoon honey
1 cup water

Combine apple cider vinegar and honey in a glass of water. Drink entire cup for rapid relief of fatigue.

Food Poisoning Prevention

Some physicians recommend this when eating questionable food sources, like when traveling to another country. This remedy can and should be used for the entire travel period as a preventative measure. If the taste of vinegar becomes too strong, honey can be added to make it more palatable.

1 tablespoon apple cider vinegar
honey (optional)

Combine apple cider vinegar with other drinking beverage (stream or tap water is not recommended, as oftentimes this may be the source of problem). Drink daily as a preventative measure 30 minutes before meals.

Flu

See "Influenza"

Foot Aches

3/4 cup apple cider vinegar
warm bath water, ankle deep

Add apple cider vinegar to warm, ankle deep bath water. Walk back and forth in water, taking care not to slip, for 5 minutes first thing in the morning, and 5 minutes in the evening before bed.

Also use this same idea to sit on the edge of the tub with your feet soaking in the water. Be sure and move your feet around as much as possible, even massaging the warm vinegar water into joints and ankle area while soaking. Press and massage into the balls of the feet for added comfort relief. Try this 2 to 3 times a day, as needed for relief.

In both cases, be sure to thoroughly dry feet when finished so you don't slip when walking.

Gas
1 teaspoon apple cider vinegar
1 cup warm water

Combine vinegar with a glass of warm water and drink slowly to end uncomfortable gas.

Headaches
1 cup apple cider vinegar
1 cup water
towel

Combine vinegar and water on the stove and bring to a boil. Pour mixture into a large bowl and place on the table. Cover head with towel, over bowl, and allow vapors to rise. Breathe in these vapors for 5 to 10 minutes to bring relief.

Headaches
1/4 cup apple cider vinegar
1/4 cup warm water

Combine apple cider vinegar and warm water and soak clean cloth. Wring out excess moisture and place on forehead and temple area. Lay in a dark room for 20 minutes.

Headaches
1/4 cup apple cider vinegar
water in vaporizer

Add vinegar to vaporizer water and inhale for 5 minutes. This works best by laying in a dark, quiet room immediately following treatment.

Headaches
apple cider vinegar
brown paper bag

Soak the bottom of the open edges of a brown paper bag in apple cider vinegar. Put the bag on the head, much like a chef's hat, and tie in place with a long scarf. Headache should be relieved in 45 minutes.

Headaches
(caused by elevated blood pressure)
2 cups apple cider vinegar
2 celery stalks, cut in half

Boil celery stalks in vinegar for 5 minutes. Remove from heat and allow to cool. At first sign of a headache caused by elevated blood pressure, chew on a vinegar-fortified celery stalk for relief.

Heartburn
See "Stomach" issues

Hiccups
1 teaspoon apple cider vinegar
1 cup warm water

Mix vinegar into glass of warm water and sip very slowly to rid hiccups.

High Blood Pressure

1 teaspoon apple cider vinegar

Some studies show that consuming a teaspoon of apple cider vinegar each day may help reduce high blood pressure.

Hives

1 tablespoon apple cider vinegar
1 tablespoon cornstarch

Blend vinegar with cornstarch into a thick paste. Use paste to blot onto itchy area and allow to completely dry. Gently wash paste off with warm water, followed by a cool rinse. Repeat as often as needed to bring relief.

Indigestion

See "Stomach" issues

Influenza

2-4 cups apple cider vinegar

Bring vinegar to a boil over medium heat. Continue to boil vinegar, uncovered, allowing vapors to permeate the entire room. After most has evaporated, use the remaining vinegar to wipe down countertops and door knobs.

Insect Bites and Stings

apple cider vinegar
cotton balls

Soak cotton ball in apple cider vinegar and gently dab over bites and stings to relieve pain and itching.

Insomnia

1 tablespoon apple cider vinegar
3/4 cup honey

Combine vinegar and honey well ahead of bedtime, so you will not later break your normal bedtime routine. About 20 minutes prior to bedtime, consume 1 teaspoon of this blend, saving the remainder for the next evening.

Insulin Spikes

1 teaspoon apple cider vinegar

Consume a teaspoon of apple cider vinegar right before meals to reduce insulin and glucose levels in the bloodstream.

Leg Cramps

1 teaspoon apple cider vinegar
1 teaspoon honey
1 tablespoon calcium lactate
3/4 cup warm water

Combine apple cider vinegar, honey and calcium lactate in a drinking glass with warm water. Drink entire solution once a day to prevent nighttime leg cramps.

Leg Cramps

1 tablespoon apple cider vinegar
1 cup water

Combine apple cider vinegar in a glass of water and drink with meals.

Muscle Aches (poultice)

1/4 cup apple cider vinegar
2 wintergreen sprigs
soft, clean cloth

Combine vinegar and sprigs together. Soak a clean cloth in vinegar solution, and apply to sore muscles for 10 minutes. Repeat as often as needed.

Muscle Aches (poultice)

1/2 cup apple cider vinegar
1/4 teaspoon cayenne pepper
soft, clean cloth

Combine vinegar and pepper in a dish. Soak soft cloth and wring out any dripping moisture. Apply to sore muscle area for 3 to 5 minutes, 3 times a day.

Nasal Congestion

1 cup apple cider vinegar
1 cup water

Combine vinegar and water in a small saucepan and bring to a boil on the stovetop. Pour vinegar solution into a bowl and place on tabletop. Cover head with towel over bowl, and breath in vapors to help reduce nasal congestion.

Nausea

See "Stomach" issues

Nosebleeds

2 teaspoons apple cider vinegar
3/4 cup water

Drink this combination daily to avoid nosebleeds.

PMS Symptoms
1 teaspoon apple cider vinegar
1 cup water

Mix apple cider vinegar and water in a glass and drink twice a day to bring relief from premenstrual symptoms.

Pneumonia
2 cups apple cider vinegar

Pour apple cider vinegar in a small pan and bring to a boil over medium heat. Boil vinegar uncovered, allowing vinegar vapors to flow throughout the room, gently breathing them in.

Shingles
2 tablespoons apple cider vinegar
2 tablespoons cornstarch

Combine vinegar and cornstarch together to form a thick paste. Gently use paste to coat painful shingle lesions by dabbing on skin and allowing it to dry completely. When needed, gently rinse with cool water and pat dry. Apply as often as needed for quick relief.

Shingles
apple cider vinegar, undiluted
clean, dry cloth

Using a soft cloth, saturate with apple cider vinegar and wring out most of the moisture. Place cloth directly over shingles for cool relief. Once used, be sure and wash the cloth in hot water to sanitize completely.

Skin Infections

apple cider vinegar
clean, dry cloth

Soak a clean, dry cloth in apple cider vinegar and wring out any excess moisture. Place vinegar-soaked cloth on body sores to heal long lasting and stubborn skin infections. Vinegar's germ-fighting ability can help eliminate bacteria on the skin and heal infection.

Sore Throat

1/4 cup apple cider vinegar
1/4 cup honey

Combine both ingredients together. Consume 1 tablespoon every 4 hours for sore throat relief. May be taken more often, if necessary.

Sore Throat

1/2 cup apple cider vinegar
1/2 cup water
1 teaspoon cayenne pepper
3 tablespoons honey

Mix all ingredients together. Keep near the bedside and sip as needed for relief.

Sore Throat

1 tablespoon white vinegar
1 cup water

Combine white vinegar and a cup of water and gargle 2 or 3 times a day for sore throat relief. Can be repeated more often, if necessary.

Sore Throat Gargle

1 tablespoon apple cider vinegar
8 ounces warm water

Mix apple cider vinegar with warm water and use as a throat gargle until sore throat has passed. Can also be used in conjunction with a drinkable sore throat for stubborn soreness.

Sprains

1 cup vinegar
bucket of hot (not boiling) water

For muscle sprains that require a hot soak, fill clean bucket with hot water (but not scalding). Add a cup of vinegar to lessen the intensity of the heat, and soak for 10 minutes on and 10 minutes off.

Sprains (poultice)

apple cider vinegar
clean, soft cloth

Soothe a sprained muscle by wrapping the sore area with a cloth wrung out of apple cider. Leave vinegar cloth in place for 5 to 7 minutes and repeat as needed.

Sprains (poultice)

1/2 cup apple cider vinegar
1/4 teaspoon cayenne pepper
soft, clean cloth

Combine vinegar and pepper in a dish. Soak soft cloth and wring out any dripping moisture. Apply to sore muscle area for 3 to 5 minutes, 3 times a day.

Sprains (poultice)
1 cup apple cider vinegar
1 tablespoon baking soda
soft, clean cloth

Combine apple cider vinegar and baking soda in a bowl. Soak a soft clean cloth in solution and wring out any excess moisture. Apply to sprain in 5 to 10 minute intervals to help reduce swelling and pain.

Stings
See "Insect Bites and Stings"

Stomach: Digestion Problems
1/2 cup apple cider vinegar
1/4 cup water
1 teaspoon fennel seeds
honey (optional)

Combine all ingredients and warm over medium heat to infuse fennel seeds. Pour into teacup and enjoy. Add dollop of honey, if desired for sweeter taste.

Stomach: Heartburn
2 teaspoons apple cider vinegar
3/4 cup water

Combine vinegar and water in a glass. Drink 10 minutes prior to eating a meal to prevent heartburn.

Stomach: Indigestion
2 cups vinegar
2 teaspoons honey
1 teaspoon fresh ginger root, grated

Combine all ingredients together. Sip after a meal that has left you with indigestion.

Stomach: Nausea

1 tablespoon apple cider vinegar
1 tablespoon honey
1 1/2 cups of water

Combine all ingredients in a drinking glass. Slowly sip on mixture to bring relief of an upset stomach.

Stomach: Nausea

2 teaspoons apple cider vinegar
2 teaspoons honey

Blend apple cider vinegar and honey and consume to end nausea.

Stomach: Nausea Poultice

1/4 cup apple cider vinegar
clean cloth

Gently warm vinegar. Soak clean cloth in warm vinegar and wring out excess moisture. Place warm vinegar cloth on stomach. As cloth cools, replace with newly warmed poultice as needed.

Sunburn

apple cider vinegar

Gently splash or spray apple cider vinegar on sunburned skin for cooling effect.

Sunburn

1/8 cup apple cider vinegar
1 cup oatmeal, cooked

Combine apple cider vinegar and cooked oatmeal to form a soft paste. Gently dab this paste onto sunburn to help ease pain and bring instant relief.

Sunburn
1/8 cup apple cider vinegar
1 teaspoon lemon juice
soft, clean cloth

Combine apple cider vinegar and lemon juice in a bowl and soak the clean cloth. Wring out any excess liquid and gently apply directly to sunburn to relieve pain.

Sunburn
1/2 cup apple cider vinegar
bath water

Pour a half cup of apple cider vinegar into cool bath water to ease the pain of sunburn and reduce the redness.

Urinary Tract Infection
1 teaspoon apple cider vinegar

Take a teaspoon of apple cider vinegar with or without water to reduce instances of urinary tract or bladder infection.

Urinary Tract Infection
1 cup apple cider vinegar
warm bath water

Add a cup of apple cider vinegar to warm bath water and soak to help bring relief of urinary tract infections.

Urinary Tract Infection
See also "Bladder Infection"

Varicose Veins
1 teaspoon apple cider vinegar
1 teaspoon honey
1 cup water

Combine one teaspoon each of apple cider vinegar and honey in a glass of water and drink once or twice a day.

Consider trying this remedy in conjunction with the vinegar poultice shown below.

Varicose Veins (Poultice)
apple cider vinegar
clean, soft cloth
honey (optional)

Soak a clean, soft cloth in undiluted apple cider vinegar. Wring out and place over varicose veins with legs propped up for 30 minutes in both the morning and evening. Considerable relief should be noticed within 6 weeks.

To speed up the healing process, follow each poultice treatment with a glass of warm water to which a teaspoon of apple cider vinegar has been added. Sip slowly and add a teaspoon of honey if feeling over tired.

Weight Loss
1 teaspoon apple cider vinegar
1 cup warm water

Mix apple cider vinegar into warm glass of water and consume before each meal. This will help moderate an over-active appetite and eliminate fat.

Welts

1 tablespoon apple cider vinegar
1 tablespoon cornstarch

Blend vinegar with cornstarch into a thick paste. Pat paste onto itchy area and allow to dry. Gently wash paste off with warm water, followed by a cool rinse.

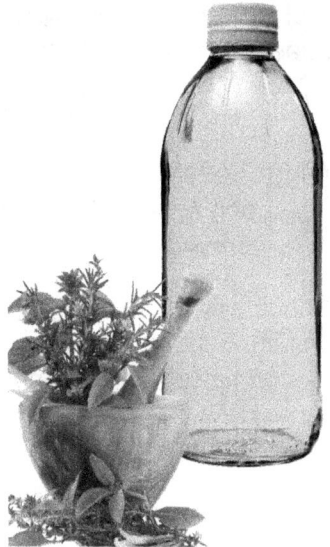

Chapter Four

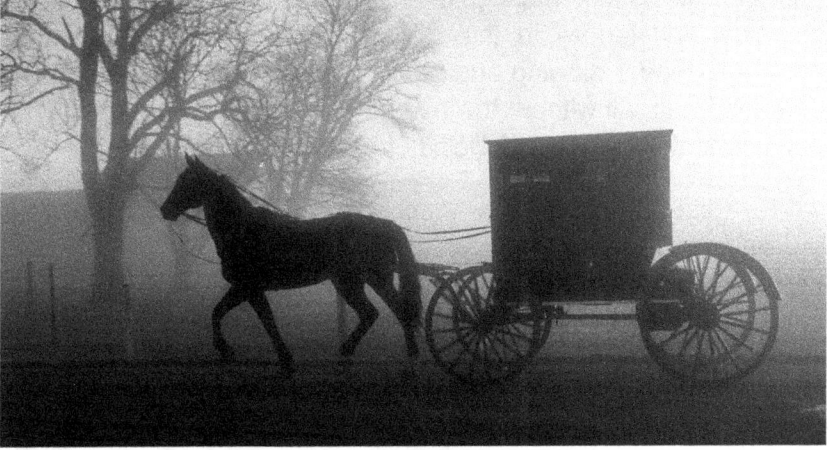

Skin Deep

Natural beauty shines through blemish-free skin and rosy cheeks of Amish women. Even after long days beneath the hot afternoon sun, their skin appears fresh and lovely.

Amish women wear no cosmetics. And while they are sometimes referred to as "plain people," they should not be confused with homely. Amish women take great care for themselves, allowing their discreet beauty to shine openly.

While the Amish do not indulge in commercial beauty products, such as makeup, expensive cleansers or the most newly touted lotions and creams, they do adhere to a wonderful beauty regimen based in nature. Likewise, Amish men are equally judicious in their use of toiletries and grooming products.

Their daily cleansing routine uses wholesome products, such as apple cider vinegar, to not only clean and nourish the skin, but also foster that radiant glow we so easily associate with them.

Apple cider vinegar has been proven to help balance pH levels in the body. Vinegar's own pH is nearly the same of that of healthy human skin tissue, making it an obvious choice to help solve chemical imbalances in the skin. Its nutrients and compounds help skin appear glowing and healthy, bring elasticity and shine to damaged hair, all without the use of harsh chemicals that can dry out skin and deplete hair follicles of essential nutrients.

Science has shown that much of the body's aging is caused by free radicals. Free radicals occur naturally as a by-product of metabolism and are responsible for degenerative diseases that come along with the aging process. They cause the skin to wrinkle, weaken the immune system and can lead to arthritis. The body's defense against these free radicals are antioxidants. And one product that can be used to help fight these free radicals through the use of antioxidants is apple cider vinegar.

Vinegar is water-soluble liquid, packed with vitamins, minerals and essential elements needed by the human body. It can help:

- Restore youthful skin

- Eliminate pimples and blemishes

- Balance pH levels in the skin

- Naturally deodorize

- Strengthen and add luster to damaged hair

- Clean and open skin pores

- Soothe and nourish dry or damaged skin

Vinegar has long been credited with the ability to act as a soothing skin tonic, add beautiful highlights to hair, and bring a calming comfort or energizing feel to the bath. Vinegar is a natural solution that the Amish have been using for generations.

Age Spots
See "Skin: Age Spots"

Armpit Odor
2-3 tablespoons apple cider vinegar
clean cloth or paper towel

Soak cloth or paper towel in undiluted apple cider vinegar. Clean armpits with vinegar cloth, but do not rinse. Allow to air dry.

Bath Soak: Herbal
Add chamomile to a vinegar bath, or substitute your favorite herbal vinegar, such as peppermint or ginger vinegar.

3/4 cup apple cider vinegar
3 tablespoons chamomile

Add vinegar and chamomile to warm bath water. Enjoy a relaxing soak for at least 20 minutes.

Bath Soak: Skin Softening
1 cup apple cider vinegar
2 herbal tea bags
warm bath water

Simmer tea bags in vinegar on stovetop for 10 minutes. Add to warm bath water for soothing, softening skin bath.

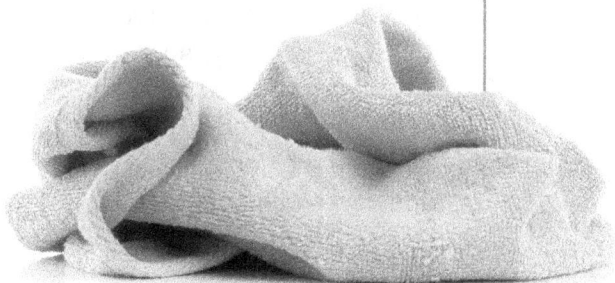

Bath Soak: Soothing
1/4 cup apple cider vinegar
2 tablespoons favorite shampoo
1 cup olive oil

Combine all ingredients together and store in a plastic bottle. Add 1/4 cup of this mixture to warm bath water for a soothing soak.

For variation, replace apple cider vinegar with tonics such as lavender or woodruff herbal vinegar.

Blackheads
See "Skin: Acne"

Body Odor
See "Armpit Odor"
See "Foot Odor"

Calluses
See "Corns and Calluses"

Corns and Calluses
1/2 cup apple cider vinegar
bucket of warm water
1 tablespoon white sugar
baby oil
mild soap

Add vinegar to bucket of warm water and soak feet for 5 minutes. Remove feet from bucket and, while still wet, rub white sugar onto bottoms of feet and any area bothered by corns or calluses. Massage sugar gently into skin. Add a bit of baby oil and continue rubbing into feet. Wash feet with mild soap and cover with cotton socks.

Denture Cleaner
Either type of vinegar can be used for this denture cleaner. White vinegar can be used, or apple cider vinegar for a more refreshing twist.

1/2 teaspoon white vinegar or apple cider vinegar
3/4 cup water

Combine your choice of vinegar and water, and allow dentures to soak overnight.

Denture Cleaner
You can also add a tablespoon of fresh mint leaves torn into pieces, to this formula for a fresh twist.

1 teaspoon white vinegar
1 cup water

Add vinegar to a cup of water. Place dentures in vinegar water and allow to soak overnight.

Denture Cleaner
Using vinegar as a brush-on denture cleaner will not only remove lingering odors, but also help brighten dentures.

1 teaspoon white vinegar
toothbrush

Brush dentures thoroughly using white vinegar. Rinse and air dry.

Deodorizer
1/4 cup apple cider vinegar
1/4 cup water

Combine both ingredients in a cup or small bowl. Following shower or bath, use to rub down high odor areas of your body, such as under the arms.

Fingernails: Beautiful Polish

Your favorite nail polish will go on smoother and stay on days longer with this quick vinegar trick.

1 teaspoon white vinegar
cotton ball

Use cotton ball to clean uncoated fingernails with vinegar and allow to air dry. Paint with favorite nail polish.

Fingernails: Fungus

1/2 cup white vinegar
1/2 cup water

Combine white vinegar and water in a shallow bowl. Soak fingernails for 10 to 15 minutes twice a day, and pat dry.

Fingernails: Fungus

white vinegar
cotton ball

Soak cotton ball with white vinegar and use to wipe down fingernails. Be sure and wipe down nails, nail bed and cuticles. Repeat 3 times a day.

Foot Odor

1 cup apple cider vinegar
1 cup warm water
1 quart strong, warm tea

Soak feet in a pan of strong, warm tea for about 5 minutes. Remove feet and rinse with warm water and apple cider vinegar. Pat dry. Can be repeated as necessary.

Foot Odor

1/4 cup apple cider vinegar
cotton balls or clean cloth

Wipe down feet twice daily with undiluted apple cider vinegar. Do not dry, but allow to air dry to remove bothersome foot odor.

Foot Softener

1/2 cup apple cider vinegar
bucket of warm water
favorite body lotion

Add vinegar to bucket of warm water. Soak feet for 10 to 15 minutes and pat dry. Apply favorite body lotion to feet and cover with a clean pair of socks.

Hair: Dandruff

2 teaspoons apple cider vinegar
1/4 cup water
comb or brush

Combine vinegar and water in a glass or bowl. Wet comb or brush in vinegar solution and brush through hair, all the way into the roots. With fingers, rub remaining vinegar solution into scalp. Allow to set 10 minutes, and then wash hair as usual.

Hair: Dandruff

1/4 cup apple cider vinegar
1/4 cup water

Combine apple cider vinegar and water in a bowl. Wash and rinse hair as usual. Follow with a second rinse of vinegar solution, but do not rinse out. Style hair as usual.

Hair: Dandruff
1/2 cup apple cider vinegar
2 cups warm water

Mix vinegar and water in a cup or bowl. Immediately after shampooing, rinse hair with vinegar mixture and style as usual.

Hair: Dandruff
1/4 cup apple cider vinegar

Wash hair as normal. For final rinse, run apple cider vinegar through hair and massage into scalp.

As a daily treatment, you can also rub vinegar into scalp and air dry without washing.

Hair: Dandruff Deep Treatment
1 cup apple cider vinegar, divided
2 crushed aspirin
1 quart warm water

Combine 1/2 cup of the vinegar and both aspirin. Wash and rinse hair as usual. Comb vinegar and aspirin solution through hair and allow to condition hair follicles for 5 minutes before rinsing completely clean. Add the second 1/2 cup of vinegar to the quart of warm water and use this as a final rinse for hair.

Hair: Frizzy and Dry
1/2 cup apple cider vinegar
1 cup warm water

Mix vinegar and warm water together in a cup. Shampoo hair as normal, and use regular conditioner. For final rinse, pour warm vinegar solution over hair and scalp. Do not rinse out.

Hair: Hair Loss

1 teaspoon apple cider vinegar
3/4 cup water

Combine vinegar and water. Drink this mixture every day for 4 to 6 weeks. New hair follicles should begin to appear after that time.

Hair: Hot Oil Treatment

1/2 cup apple cider vinegar
1/4 cup olive oil
hot water

Heat olive oil until warm and massage into hair. Allow more oil on strands of hair and into hair ends, avoiding a lot of oil getting into the scalp. Fill a sink or bowl with hot tap water and add vinegar. Soak a bath towel in vinegar water and wring it out by hand. Wrap the wet, warm towel around hair, and allow to soak in for 20 to 30 minutes. Remove towel and wash hair as normal. Repeat every month, or more often for particularly dry or damaged hair.

Hair: Moisturizer

1/2 apple cider vinegar, divided
2 teaspoons honey
1 egg yolk
1/3 cup olive oil
bath towel

Combine all ingredients except 1/4 cup of the vinegar; set that aside. Gently rub mixture into hair and scalp 10 minutes before washing. Wrap treated hair in towel and allow to penetrate for 10 minutes. Shampoo as usual, and rinse in lukewarm water with final 1/4 cup of apple cider vinegar.

Hair: Maintain Richness

4 teaspoons apple cider vinegar
4 teaspoons black strap molasses
4 teaspoons honey
1 cup water

Mix all ingredients together in a large glass. Begin each day by drinking this concoction to maintain a rich, healthy head of hair.

Hair: Rinse

1/2 cup apple cider vinegar
1/4 cup water

Combine both ingredients together. Following a shower or bath, give hair a final rinse with vinegar water solution. Do not rinse out, but instead allow to air dry.

Hands: Hand Softener

1 teaspoon vinegar
1/2 cup water
1/2 teaspoon white sugar
1 teaspoon baby oil

Crudely combine all ingredients and then pour over hands. Work this mixture into hands for 2 minutes, covering all parts of hands including backs, palms and between fingers. Wash clean with a mild soap. Use daily or as needed.

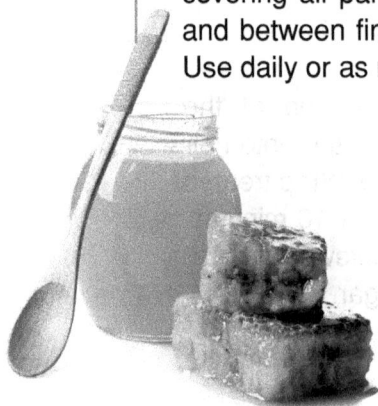

Hands: Hand Softener

1 tablespoon apple cider vinegar
2 cups warm water
1/2 teaspoon petroleum jelly
clean cotton gloves
soft cloth or towel

Add vinegar to warm water and soak hands for 5 minutes. Pat hands dry with a soft cloth or towel. Smooth petroleum jelly over hands and cover with clean cotton gloves. Wear gloves overnight. By morning hands will be unbelievably soft and smooth.

Hands: Soiled

1 tablespoon white or apple cider vinegar
1 teaspoon cornmeal

Wet soiled hands with vinegar. Sprinkle cornmeal into both hands and rub vigorously together. Rinse in cool water and pat dry.

Liver Spots

See "Skin: Age Spots"

Mouthwash

Both types of vinegars are recommended here. Apple cider vinegar can be used for any healing that needs to take place in the mouth. White vinegar can be used for a more intense flavor.

2 tablespoons apple cider vinegar or white vinegar
1/8 teaspoon peppermint flavoring (not oil)
1 cup warm water

Add your choice of vinegar and peppermint flavoring to a glass of warm water. Gargle and rinse mouth clean.

pH Levels
See "Skin: pH Levels"

Pimples
See "Skin: Acne"

Rectal Itching
1/8 cup apple cider vinegar
thick gauze square

Soak clean gauze in apple cider vinegar and apply directly to itch for instant relief. Repeat as needed.

Skin: Acne
1 teaspoon apple cider vinegar
1 teaspoon honey
1 tablespoon cornstarch

Combine ingredients together to form a thick paste. Use paste on pimples and blackheads by gently rubbing solution into blemishes in a circular motion.

Skin: Age Spots
2 teaspoons apple cider vinegar
1 teaspoon onion juice

Combine apple cider vinegar and onion juice and apply with a soft cloth or piece of cotton to age spots.

Skin: Age Spots
1 tablespoon apple cider vinegar
1/2 onion

Dab the cut side of the onion into vinegar and rub gently directly onto age spots once a day. Age spots should begin to fade in a few weeks.

Skin: Facial
1 cup apple cider vinegar
clean towel

Heat cup of vinegar and bring to a boil. Remove vinegar from stove and carefully pour hot vinegar into a large bowl. Lean over the bowl using the towel to cover your head over the bowl. Allow the warm steam to soften facial skin. Remain with face over bowl until steaming action has ended.

After vinegar has cooled and you are no longer able to use it for steaming, gently dab a little of the vinegar onto the face as a cleaning astringent.

Skin: Facial
1/2 cup apple cider vinegar
1/4 cup oatmeal
1/4 cup cooked rice

Combine all ingredients in a medium bowl until thoroughly mixed. Pat mixture onto face and neck and allow to dry for about 10 minutes. Wash off paste with lukewarm water. Rinse with cool water and gently pat skin dry with a clean, soft towel.

Skin: Facial
1 tablespoon apple cider vinegar
1 tablespoon honey
1/2 mashed banana
1/2 mashed peach

Combine all ingredients in a bowl until a sticky paste forms. Gently apply to neck and face and allow to set for about 10 minutes. Rinse clean and pat dry.

Skin: Facial Mask Moisturizer

1 tablespoon apple cider vinegar
1 tablespoon honey
1/4 cup oatmeal

Mix all ingredients until well blended. Gently pat mixture onto wet facial skin and allow to air dry. Rinse off with cool water and apply favorite moisturizer.

Skin: Facial Toner

1/2 cup apple cider vinegar
1/2 cup water
plastic bottle
cotton balls

Combine vinegar and water and pour into a plastic bottle. Use cotton ball to apply daily to face and neck.

Skin: Itchy Skin

3 cups apple cider vinegar
warm bath water
handful of thyme (optional)

Fill bathtub with warm water and add apple cider vinegar. Sprinkle handful of thyme in the water, if desired, and soak in vinegar bath once a day to relieve all-over dry, itchy skin.

Skin: Lightening

1/4 cup white vinegar
1/4 cup lemon juice
1/2 cup white wine
1 tablespoon honey

Combine ingredients and mix until well incorporated. Store in a jar or bottle. Twice a day, gently apply solution to face by blotting on with a soft cotton ball.

Skin: Men's After Shave

Great herbs for men's after shave are thyme, sage, bay leaves or cloves. Also add bee balm, chamomile and spearmint.

1 cup white vinegar
2 tablespoon honey
1 tablespoon favorite herb

Combine all ingredients together and place in a small jar with a tight fitting lid. Allow to rest undisturbed for up to one week. Open jar and strain out any floating herbs or debris. Daily aftershave is now ready for use.

Skin: Men's After Shave Cooler

1 cup white vinegar
2 tablespoons honey
1 small cucumber
mint leaves

Place cucumber with peel in a blender along with fresh mint leaves. Puree into a fine mixture. Combine all ingredients, including cucumber, in a small jar and seal with lid. Place in refrigerator overnight. Strain out any cucumber peel or floating herbs using a sieve. Pour tonic into a glass or plastic decanter, preferably one using a pump action dispenser. Use daily.

Skin: Men's Skin Bracer

2 tablespoons white vinegar
1/2 teaspoon cream of tartar
1/3 cup warm water

Combine all ingredients together. Wash face and pat dry. Gently pat bracer onto skin.

Skin: pH Level Balancing
2 teaspoons apple cider vinegar
clean cloth or towelette

Soak a clean cloth or towelette in apple cider vinegar.
Gently apply to face daily to balance skin's pH levels.

Skin: pH Level Balancing Body Wash
This body wash is a great way to help balance the
body's pH levels

1/2 cup apple cider vinegar
1/2 cup water

Combine both ingredients together and use to splash
on your body after bathing. Solution will leave your
skin silky soft as it balances pH levels and frees skin
from drying soap.

Skin: Prevent Outdoor Dryness
1/4 cup apple cider vinegar
1/4 cup olive oil

Mix apple cider vinegar and olive oil and apply a
protective coating to exposed skin before going
outdoors. This extra moisturizer will help prevent
chapping.

Skin: Radiant Skin
1/4 cup vinegar
3 large strawberries

Mash strawberries into vinegar and let set
undisturbed for 2 hours. Strain strawberry-vinegar
solution though a cloth or sieve and discard lumps.
Before bed, pat strawberry flavored vinegar onto
face and neck. In the morning, wash solution off face
with normal morning cleansing routine.

Skin: Wrinkles
1 cup apple cider vinegar
1 tablespoon fennel seeds

Combine vinegar and fennel seeds and heat over medium heat until hot. Turn the heat down and allow to simmer for 30 minutes, uncovered, allowing some of the moisture to evaporate out. Remove from heat and cool completely. Pour into a jar with a tight-fitting lid.

Saturate a cotton ball with fennel-infused vinegar and gently dab over face and neck. For even greater soothing action, gently heat jar of fennel vinegar in microwave before using. Use warm vinegar and fennel combination to dab over wrinkles, allowing for greater moisturizing penetration.

Use once or twice a day.

Sunburn
apple cider vinegar, undiluted
clean cloth

Saturate a clean cloth with apple cider vinegar. Gently place cloth on sunburned area of skin for instant relief.

Sunburn Soak
1 cup apple cider vinegar
lukewarm bathtub of water

Fill bathtub with lukewarm water, taking care to not allow temperature to become too hot. Add vinegar and soak for 15 to 20 minutes for relief of sunburn pain.

Toenails: Trimming

Try this to soften nails immediately prior to trimming.

3 tablespoons apple cider vinegar
4 cups warm water

Combine vinegar and warm water. Soak feet and toes in solution for 10 minutes, right before trimming nails. Dry feet and proceed to trim toe nails.

Warts

1 teaspoon apple cider vinegar
small cotton gauze or cotton ball
tape

Soak piece of cotton gauze or cotton ball in vinegar. Place soaked cotton ball on wart and tape into place. Leave on wart for 30 minutes. Repeat twice a day until wart is gone.

Weight Loss

2 teaspoons apple cider vinegar
1 cup water

Stir apple cider vinegar into a glass of water. Drink full glass of vinegar water 20 minutes before mealtime to suppress appetite and stimulate weight loss.

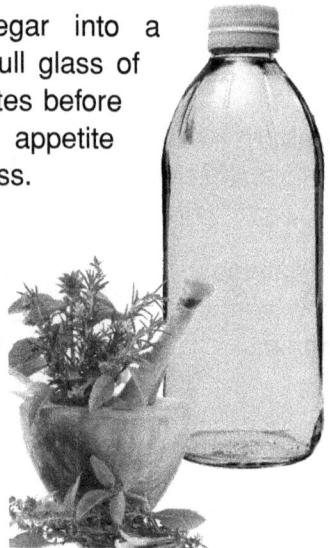

Chapter Five

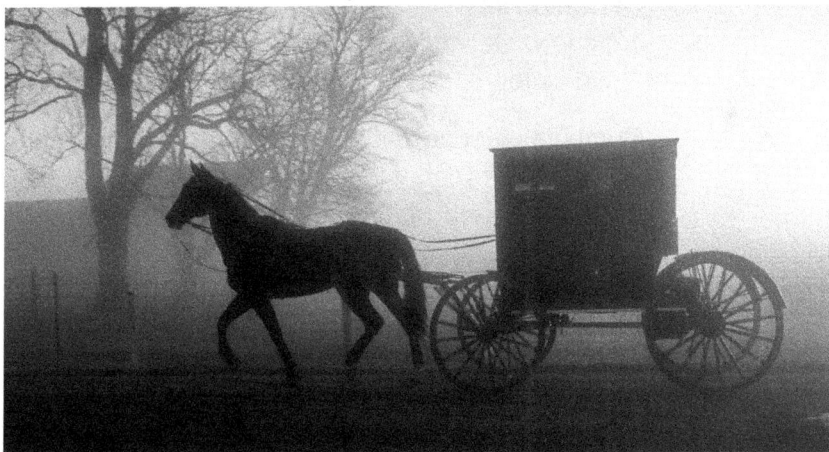

Amish Clean

Amish women take seriously their privilege of keeping a lovely family home. They relish in being good homemakers, providing a comfortable and welcoming home for all who enter. Kitchens are kept clean, common areas are uncluttered and inviting.

One would expect to see film build-up in kitchens from years of kerosene cook stove use, or evidence of creosote after generations of reliance on wood burning stoves. But Amish homes are some of the cleanest you will find. And they keep homes clean through the use of natural cleaning products, instead of many commercial cleaning solutions.

Benefits of using natural disinfecting substances, like vinegar, mean the avoidance of harmful toxins and chemical residues. Vinegar is 100% natural and save for both children and pets.

Some of the very best natural cleaning regimens come from Amish homes, where they have been tested over time and passed down for generations.

Ceramic Tile
1/4 cup white vinegar
1 cup water

Combine vinegar and water. Use a cloth or sponge to wipe down ceramic tile in the bathroom to keep soap scum and hard water deposits from building up. Dry thoroughly with a clean towel.

Exhaust Fans
white vinegar, undiluted

Wipe and clean exhaust fan grill cover, removing dust and debris. Using a clean cloth wet with vinegar, wipe down grill cover coating it with vinegar to keep dust from accumulating on fan grill.

Fixtures: Chrome and Brass
1/2 cup white vinegar
2 cups warm water
wax

In sink or small bucket, combine vinegar and water. Using a soft cloth, clean chrome and brass. Dry completely. Apply two coats of a light wax to coat and shine. Coating will make future bathroom fixture clean up easier and prevent build up of hard water deposits.

Mirrors
white vinegar, undiluted
soft, clean cloth

Spray vinegar directly onto clean cloth. Use cloth to wipe mirror into a streak-free shine. Do not spray vinegar, or any other solution, directly onto mirror. Moisture can make its way into silver backing and destroy mirror.

Odors
1 tablespoon white vinegar
1/2 cup water
small spray bottle

Fill a small spray bottle with vinegar and water. Use a few sprays of this natural deodorizer in the place of aerosol air fresheners.

Shower Curtains
2 cups white vinegar
warm water to cover curtain
2 tablespoons liquid dish detergent

Remove shower curtain from hooks and place in bathtub or wash tub. Fill tub with just enough water to completely cover shower curtain. Pour in 2 cups of white vinegar. Allow shower curtain to soak in vinegar water at least 4 hours, or overnight if possible.

In the morning, add liquid detergent to vinegar water and wash curtain in tub. Rinse curtain and hang outside to dry in the afternoon sun.

Shower Doors, Glass
1/4 cup white vinegar
1 teaspoon alum

Mix white vinegar and alum together. Wipe mixture on glass shower door and scrub with a soft cleaning brush. Rinse with hot water. Buff with a soft cloth until completely dry.

Shower Doors, Mildew

white vinegar, undiluted
water
old toothbrush
cleaning cloth
spray bottle

Dip old toothbrush into undiluted vinegar and use to scrub out corners and crevices of shower door. Fill spray bottle with white vinegar and use to thoroughly wet shower door. Wipe clean with a cloth saturated in vinegar.

Shower Head

white vinegar, undiluted
paper towels
plastic bag
rubber band
scrub brush

Soak paper towels in vinegar until fully saturated. Wrap saturated paper towels tightly against the shower head. Do not wring out paper towels. Place plastic bag around coated shower head and secure with a rubber band. Leave to soak overnight.

In the morning, remove plastic bag and paper towels and discard. Use a scrub brush with additional vinegar and brush away any remaining mineral scales.

Shower Head

1/2 cup white vinegar
2/3 cup water

Combine vinegar and water. Use soft cleaning brush to scrub clean mineral build up on bathroom shower heads.

Shower Head
white vinegar, undiluted
hot rinse water
cleaning brush
toothpick or nail
toothbrush

Unscrew shower head and place in sink with enough undiluted white vinegar to cover shower head. Allow to soak for 30-45 minutes, more if necessary. Remove shower head and gently brush with a cleaning brush. Use toothpick or nail to clean out small openings, if blocked. Scrub around openings with an old toothbrush. Rinse in hot water. Dry to a shine with a buffing towel and replace.

Toilet Stains
1 cup white vinegar
1 cup borax

Pour vinegar over stained porcelain toilet. Sprinkle borax over wet vinegar stain and let soak for 2 hours. Brush with a toilet brush and flush away.

Soap Scum Removal
1/2 cup white vinegar, divided
1/2 cup ammonia
3 tablespoons baking soda

Combine 1/2 cup white vinegar, ammonia and baking soda, and stir into a thick paste. Spread paste over soap scum and allow to set for at least 10 minutes. Gently scrub with a cleaning brush. Rinse with a bucket of cool water to which 1/4 cup of additional vinegar has been added. After removing soap scum from shower and door, use Soap Film Preventative (next page) to keep from returning.

Soap Film Preventative

Use this solution as a preventative from soap film and scum in bathroom showers and tubs.

1 cup white vinegar
1 quart water
spray bottle

Fill spray bottle with vinegar and water. Once a week, spray down shower and tub area to prevent soap film from building up in tub area.

Soap Film Removal

1/2 cup white vinegar, plus 1/4 cup white vinegar
1 cup baking soda
water

In a bowl, combine vinegar and baking soda into a creamy paste, adding additional vinegar if needed. Spread paste over soap film in shower and allow to set for 10 minutes. Use a soft brush to clean film. Rinse with warm bucket of water to which 1/4 cup vinegar has been added. Use a soft cloth to buff dry.

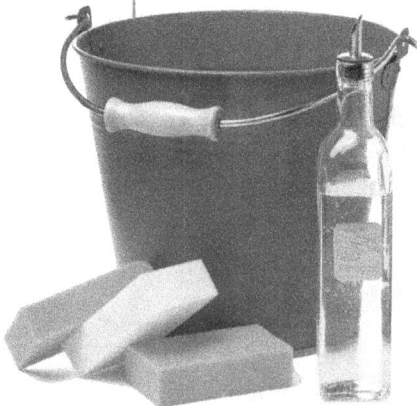

In The Kitchen

Appliances

1/4 cup white vinegar
1 teaspoon borax
2 cups hot water
plastic spray bottle

Combine ingredients and pour into spray bottle. Spray vinegar solution on greasy smears on kitchen appliances. Buff in a circular motion with a soft cloth.

Appliances: Black

Black or dark colored appliances, like stainless steel, seem to show every fingerprint or smudge. They also tend to show swirl markings from cleaning. Try this formula to keep black appliances looking new and smudge free.

white vinegar, undiluted
soft, lint-free cloth

Clean appliance as usual. Using undiluted vinegar on a soft, lint-free cloth, do a final wipe down of the appliance. Buff with a clean cloth.

Appliances: Can Openers

white vinegar, undiluted
cotton swabs
bowl
soft cloth

Wipe down can opener with a soft cloth dipped in vinegar. Soak removable opener blade in a small bowl of white vinegar to remove encrusted food; carefully wipe clean. Use a vinegar-soaked cotton swab tip to clean can opener vents and operation buttons. Wipe dry with a clean cloth.

Appliances: Coffee Pots
1 tablespoon white vinegar
water

Fill coffee pot with water and add white vinegar. Allow to set for 10 minutes, and rinse well.

Appliances: Coffee Pots
1 cup white vinegar
1 cup water

Combine white vinegar and water. Run this solution through an automatic coffee pot brewing cycle.

Kitchen: Coffee Pots
1 tablespoon white vinegar
2-3 drops dish detergent
water

In coffee receptacle, pour vinegar and detergent. Run one pot of water through full brewing cycle. Rinse pot several times with hot water.

Appliances: Dishwashers
When cleaning automatic dishwashers, be careful not to completely dry inside bottom of appliance. Some manufacturers depend on a small amount of moisture to keep seals from drying out and cracking.

2 cups white vinegar
cleaning rag

Pour undiluted vinegar into bottom of empty dishwasher. Run dishwasher without using any detergent, only the vinegar. When both wash and rinse cycles end, but before drying cycle begins, turn off dishwasher and wipe down the interior top, sides and door with a cleaning cloth.

Appliances: Electric Knives
white vinegar, undiluted
few drops liquid dish detergent
soft cloth
toothpick

Wipe electric knife with a cloth dampened with vinegar and soapy water. Saturate area around dirty blade mounting, and set for 5 minutes. Use toothpick to scrape area clean. Wipe electric cord and dry thoroughly.

Appliances: Exhaust Fan Grill
white vinegar, undiluted
clean cloth

Wash exhaust fan grill, removing any dust and debris. Wet clean cloth with vinegar and wipe down fan grill to remove any remaining grease. This will help retard grease build up in the future.

Appliances: Garbage Disposal
1/2 cup white vinegar
ice cubes

Run a tray of ice cubes down the garbage disposal with 1/2 cup white vinegar poured over them each week for a fresh disposal.

Appliances: Microwave Ovens
3 tablespoons apple cider vinegar
1 cup water

Pour vinegar and water into a microwave-safe cup or bowl. Bring vinegar mixture to a boil in the microwave and allow to set in closed microwave for 5 minutes. Microwave will smell fresh and vinegar-clean.

Appliances: Microwave Ovens

1/2 cup white vinegar
1/2 cup water

In a small, microwave-safe bowl, heat vinegar and water in the microwave until it begins to boil. Now run the microwave on its highest setting for 30 seconds. Spills and baked-on foods should now wipe down with ease.

For any additional cleaning, use a clean cloth and the rest of the vinegar solution (once it cools) to wipe away grime.

Appliances: Mixers

white vinegar
soft cleaning cloth

Saturate clean cloth with vinegar and wrap cloth around mixer. Allow to set for 5 minutes. Remove vinegar-soaked cloth and wipe clean.

Appliances: Oven

1 cup vinegar, plus extra for spraying
1 tablespoon dish detergent
tub of hot water
spray bottle

Remove racks from oven and spray thoroughly with vinegar (you may wish to do this outdoors). Allow racks to air dry. Place racks in tub of very hot water, vinegar and dish detergent. Let racks to soak for 30 minutes. Turn racks and repeat on opposite end if you are unable to fit entire rack in tub at one time. You may need to soak racks a second time. Wipe down racks with a cloth or sponge.

Appliances: Oven

When using ammonia, you may wish to use rubber or plastic cleaning gloves to protect your hands.

1/2 cup white vinegar
3 cups water
2 cups ammonia
2 cups baking soda

Pour water into a shallow baking dish and place in oven. Heat oven to 300°. Turn off oven and allow water to remain in warm oven for 30 minutes. After 30 minutes, remove baking dish and discard water. Replace with ammonia and put back in warm oven (keeping oven turned off) and allow to set overnight.

In the morning, pour all out except 1/2 cup of ammonia. Add white vinegar and baking soda to remaining ammonia. Use this mixture to wash down oven surfaces and then allow to set on oven surfaces for 30 minutes. After 30 minutes, wipe away oven cleaner and rinse with clean water. Dry.

Appliances: Refrigerators

Use this to remove any dirt or grease layer that has built up on the top of your refrigerator.

white vinegar, undiluted
few drops liquid detergent
spray bottle

Spray undiluted vinegar on top of refrigerator and add a few drops of liquid detergent. Using a cloth or sponge, give the entire appliance top a quick pat to make sure vinegar and detergent is in contact with any grease build up. Allow to soak for 15 minutes. Wipe clean with cloth or sponge. Rinse with hot water and a tablespoon or two of additional vinegar, and dry completely.

Appliances: Refrigerators and Freezer Gaskets
white vinegar, undiluted
1 teaspoon liquid detergent
2 cups warm water

Squirt liquid detergent into water and use to wipe down refrigerator and freezer gaskets. Use undiluted vinegar to wipe away any mold. Rinse and dry with a clean towel.

Appliances: Refrigerators, Self-Defrosting
1 tablespoon white vinegar
few drops liquid detergent

Remove water collecting tray and wash in hot, soapy water. Dry tray and replace. Add vinegar to water collecting tray to retard growth of bacteria and keep refrigerator fresh.

Appliances: Small Appliances
When cleaning any small appliances, be sure not to spray any liquid solution directly onto the appliance. Keep moisture from entering the appliance's vent to protect internal parts from damage. Appliances should always be unplugged prior to cleaning.

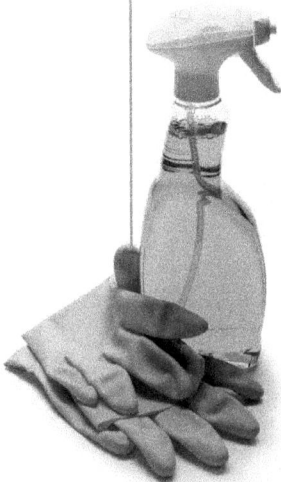

White vinegar, undiluted
clean cloths

Wipe down appliance with clean cloth saturated with white vinegar. Use a second clean cloth to buff appliance dry.

Appliances: Small Appliance Buttons
white vinegar, undiluted
cotton swabs

Saturate tip of a cotton swab with vinegar. Use to clean tops and around sides of appliance buttons and control knobs.

Appliances: Small Appliance Cords
white vinegar, undiluted
soft cloths

Wet a soft cloth with vinegar. Use to periodically wipe down appliance cords to keep free from food and other debris. Dry with another soft cloth.

Appliances: Stove Tops
1/2 cup white vinegar
1/2 cup water
1 teaspoon liquid detergent

Combine all ingredients together. Using a soft cloth, wipe down stove tops to rid cooked on food and grease. Rinse clean with a cloth wet with water and buff dry.

Appliances: Stove Tops, Gas Grates
1 cup white vinegar
2 cups water

On a stove top, place individual iron grates from gas stove in a pot of vinegar and water. Bring to a boil for 10 minutes. Remove from vinegar water and wipe clean.

Countertop
white vinegar

Wipe down all kitchen countertops and work surfaces with undiluted white vinegar to clean, disinfect and prevent mold.

Countertop Cleaner
1 cup white vinegar
1 cup water
spray bottle

Combine vinegar and water and store in a plastic spray bottle. Use this solution to wipe down kitchen countertops, as needed.

Make a bottleful of this natural cleaner ahead of time to keep on hand each time you clean the kitchen.

Countertop Cleaner
Keep this scrubber on hand for easy cleaning that will not damage countertop surfaces.

White vinegar, undiluted
discarded nylon hosiery

Completely soak nylon hosiery in undiluted white vinegar. Use to scrub hard-to-clean areas of kitchen countertops.

Countertop Cleaner, Hard to Clean
white vinegar, undiluted
paper towels

Soak a paper towel in undiluted white vinegar. Lay the soaked paper towel on the caked area and allow to set for 30 to 60 minutes. Wipe clean.

Countertop Disinfectant

3 tablespoons white vinegar
1 teaspoon liquid soap
1/2 teaspoon oil
1/2 cup water

Combine all ingredients. Using a wash towel, wipe down kitchen counters to thoroughly disinfect.

Countertop Stain Remover

1/4 cup white vinegar
1/4 cup water

Combine white vinegar and water together and use to wipe down stained counter. For more difficult stains, allow cloth soaked in this solution to lay on top of the stain for 15 minutes before wiping clean.

Cutting Boards and Cutting Blocks

apple cider vinegar, undiluted

Wipe down wood cutting boards with undiluted apple cider vinegar to clean, disinfect and absorb any lingering odors.

Cutting Boards and Cutting Blocks

white vinegar, undiluted
1 tablespoon baking soda
plastic spray bottle

Sprinkle baking soda over wooden cutting board or block and gently rub into wood. Spray baking soda with undiluted white vinegar and allow to stand for 5 minutes. Rinse with clean water, allowing solution to bubble. Rinse and wipe away any remaining solution.

Cutting Boards, Deep Sanitation
1/2 cup white vinegar
2-3 tablespoons salt
2 teaspoons vegetable oil (for wood cutting boards)

Apply salt to coat cutting board (use more if necessary) and allow to rest for 10 minutes. Scrub salt with a vinegar wash and rinse well using hot water. Dry with a cloth. For wood cutting boards, occasionally rub in vegetable oil to keep wood like new.

Deodorizer
apple cider vinegar, undiluted
clean cloth

Soak a clean cloth in apple cider vinegar and wring out any excess moisture. Place wet cloth on top of heat or air register and allow air to circulate through moistened cloth for 30 minutes to make kitchen smell fresh and odor free.

Deodorizer
2 tablespoons white vinegar
4 ounce pump bottle

Fill pump bottle with vinegar, After cooking fish, cabbage or for boil overs, spray a few pumps of undiluted vinegar in the air to neutralize odor.

Deodorizer, Eliminate Cooking Odors
1/4 cup white or apple cider vinegar
1 teaspoon cinnamon

Simmer vinegar in an uncovered pot of water to clear the air of lingering cooking odors. For a clean smell, use white vinegar; for a special air freshened scent, use apple cider vinegar with cinnamon added.

Drains

1/2 cup white vinegar

Pour undiluted vinegar down each drain weekly to keep drains fresh and discourage clogging. No need to rinse away.

Drains

This is a great drain cleaning solution to freshen and open up slow moving kitchen drains.

1/2 cup white vinegar
1/2 cup baking soda
hot water

Pour baking soda down drain. Follow baking soda with undiluted white vinegar and allow to rest in drain for 10 minutes. Run hot water down drain to rinse clean.

Drains and Septics

Use this solution once a month to keep drains running free and give a bacteria boost to septic systems. It also will help cleanse lingering odors.

Drain cleaner solution above
1 package dry yeast
2/3 cup brown sugar

Using drain cleaning solution above, treat each drain in the house. After treating drains, proceed to also treat septic tank by pouring yeast and brown sugar into toilet and flushing tank twice.

Doing this monthly will help keep the drain and septic system running efficiently for many years.

Faucets and Fixtures
1 tablespoon white vinegar
1 tablespoon cream of tartar
warm water
clean cloth

Mix ingredients into a paste. Rub paste onto dingy faucets and kitchen fixtures and allow to dry completely. Using a pan of warm water, wash dried paste off all fixtures and buff dry with a clean cloth.

Faucets and Fixtures
1/3 cup white vinegar
2/3 cup water

Combine vinegar and water. Use a soft cloth to polish and shine faucets and fixtures.

Garbage Disposal
Freshen disposals with this weekly treatment.

1/2 cup white vinegar
tray of ice cubes

Dump tray of ice cubes down kitchen drain. Pour vinegar over cubes. Run water over ice and vinegar while running garbage disposal to clean and freshen.

Garbage Disposal
1/2 cup vinegar
1/2 cup water

Combine vinegar and water and fill ice cube tray. Freeze cubes. Frozen vinegar cubes can be stored in a plastic zip bag in the freezer for future use.

Grind a handful of these vinegar cubes in the garbage disposal each week to keep disposal blades sharp and disposal system odor free.

Dishes: Aluminum Pots and Pans

1/2 cup white vinegar
2 cups water

Pour vinegar and water into aluminum pan. Bring to a boil. Pour out solution and wipe pan clean.

Dishes: Aluminum Pots and Pans Stains

1 tablespoon white vinegar
1 teaspoon baking soda

Combine vinegar and baking soda into a paste. Use this paste to clean, using a circular motion, light stains from aluminum cookware.

Dishes: Aluminum Pots and Pans Stains

Try this solution for heavy and hard to clean stains.

1 tablespoon white vinegar
1 teaspoon baking soda
1 teaspoon cream of tartar

Combine all three ingredients and mix into a paste. Rubbing in a circular motion, remove stains from aluminum cooking pots and pans.

Dishes: Aluminum Pots and Pans Stains

Another solution for heavily stained pots and pans

1 tablespoon white vinegar
1 teaspoon liquid dish detergent
1 teaspoon baking soda
1 teaspoon cream of tartar
nylon scrubbing pad

Combine ingredients together to form a gritty gel. Spread gel over stains in pan and rub in a circular motion with nylon scrubbing pad to remove stains. Rinse well. Repeat a second time, if necessary.

Dishes: Ceramic Baking Dishes
1/8 cup white vinegar
nylon scrubber

Pour vinegar in a small bowl. Use nylon scrubber to remove baked on food from ceramic bakeware. Wash as usual.

Dishes: Copper and Brass Cleaner
1/4 cup white vinegar
1/4 cup lemon juice
paper towel
soft cloth

Combine both ingredients in a small bowl. Apply mixture to copper or brass with a paper towel. Buff to a beautiful shine with a soft cloth.

Dishes: Copper Pan Cleaner
1 cup white vinegar
1/2 cup powdered dish detergent
1/2 cup water
1/2 cup salt
1/4 cup flour

Mix all ingredients in a bowl, whisking until thoroughly blended. Heat slowly in a double boiler until detergent is dissolved and mixture begins to thicken. Remove from heat and cool completely. Once cool, use this mixture to wipe onto a copper pot and coat. Allow to set for 1 minute, and wipe clean with a soft cloth.

Dishes: Enamel Baking Dishes
2 cups white vinegar

Wash all easy-to-remove food from enamel baking dish. Pour in vinegar to cover baked on food. If 2 cups is not enough, add more as needed. Place baking dish on stovetop or in oven and bring vinegar to a boil in baking dish. Boil for several minutes before removing from heat and allow to cool. Pour out vinegar and wash baking dish as usual.

Dishes: Fine China
Fine china should be washed by hand. Note: This solution is for china that is free from gold or silver trim. Vinegar is known to cause metal trim work to discolor.

1/4 cup white vinegar
water
liquid dish detergent
paper plates or paper towels

Gently wash fine china by hand in warm, soapy water. Rinse in sink full of hot water and vinegar. Dry each piece of china with a clean, soft cloth. To store safely, place a paper plate or paper towel between each piece of china to prevent chipping.

Dishes: Glassware
1/4 cup white vinegar
hot rinse water

Add vinegar to final rinse water. After cleaning, soak glassware in hot vinegar water. Remove and allow to air dry.

Dishes: Grease Cutter
1/2 cup white vinegar
warm to hot dishwater

Add vinegar to dishwater, using your favorite dish soap as usual. Vinegar will work to cut heavy grease in the water for cleaner dishes.

Dishes: Lead Crystal

Lead crystal should always be washed by hand, never in the dishwasher.

1/4 cup white vinegar
liquid dish detergent
water

Make a sink full of warm, soapy water with liquid detergent. Place a rubber tub mat in bottom of sink to keep lead crystal safe from chips and scratches. Submerge lead crystal into soapy water and wash thoroughly. Rinse in sink full of hot water and white vinegar. Place crystal on clean towel or drying rack to air dry.

Dishes: Musty Glass Jars

white vinegar, undiluted
clean sponge

Dampen a clean sponge with vinegar and wring out any excess. Place dampened sponge in jar and seal tightly with lid. Leave to soak up musty odors for at least 1 hour.

Dishes: Non-Stick Pans

This solution will help remove mineral deposits and other stains from non-stick coated cookware without damaging the coating.

1/3 cup white vinegar
2 cups water

Pour water and vinegar into non-stick pan stained with mineral deposits. Bring to a boil over medium heat on stovetop. Allow to boil for 3 to 5 minutes. Discard solution and wipe pan clean with a soft cloth.

Dishes: Pewter
3 tablespoons white vinegar
cabbage leaves
1 teaspoon salt

Soak cabbage leaves in vinegar. Dip wet cabbage leaf in salt, and use to buff pewter. Rinse with cool water and dry pewter.

Dishes: Pewter
1 tablespoon white vinegar
1 tablespoon salt
1 tablespoon flour

Combine vinegar, salt and flour together using just enough vinegar to form a paste. Smear paste on discolored pewter and allow to dry completely. Rub off the dried paste. Rinse in hot water and buff completely dry.

Dishes: Greasy Pots and Pans
white vinegar, undiluted
spray bottle

Place undiluted vinegar in a spray bottle. Spray a thick coat of vinegar on greasy pots. Allow to sit 3-5 minutes. Grease will come off easier, using less dish soap.

Dishes: Stuck on Food
1/2 cup white vinegar
1 1/2 cups water

Combine vinegar and water and add to pots with stuck on food. Heat vinegar and water mixture in dirty pot, and wipe clean.

Dishes: Thermoses

1 cup white vinegar
1/2 cup water
1 tablespoon rice, uncooked

Combine vinegar and water and use it to fill thermos. Fit with lid and shake to coat entire inside of thermos. Let stand for 1 hour. After an hour, add uncooked rice and shake for an additional 2 minutes. Pour out contents and rinse thoroughly. Wipe dry.

Dishes: Vases

Odd shaped flower vases can be difficult to clean due to their shape and narrow openings.

1/8 cup white vinegar
nylon scrub brush

Pour vinegar into small dish. Use nylon scrub brush dipped in white vinegar to clean hard-to-reach areas of the vase interior. Rinse with hot water and air dry.

Dishes: Vases

1/2 cup white vinegar, plus 1/4 cup white vinegar
1/4 cup uncooked rice
1/2 cup cold water
1/3 cup warm water

Pour uncooked rice into vase opening. Follow rice with 1/2 cup white vinegar and cold water. Shake vase, spinning it in a circular motion, then in reverse direction to loosen dirt or grime. Let set for 1 minute, and repeat shaking and swirling action. Pour out rice and vinegar solution. Rinse out vase with 1/4 cup white vinegar and warm water. Empty contents and set upside down on countertop to allow to air dry.

Dishes: Vases

1/4 cup white vinegar
1/4 cup hot water
3 tablespoons sand

Pour sand into vase opening. Follow with vinegar and hot water. Shake or swirl vase vigorously, removing dirt deposits from inside of vase. Empty all contents from vase and rinse well before drying.

Dishes: Vases

white vinegar, undiluted
paper towel

Soak paper towel with undiluted white vinegar and use to wipe down inside of vase to remove lingering waterlines.

Floors: Carpet Cleaning

As with any new cleaning method, be sure to test a small area of the carpet for colorfastness before cleaning larger areas.

1 cup white vinegar
1 gallon water

Combine white vinegar and water together and pour into a spray bottle. Spray carpet in areas that need cleaned, saturating carpet and allowing to soak in for several minutes. Wipe clean with an absorbent cloth or towel. If stain is persistent, repeat a second time, doing so before carpet has had an opportunity to dry.

Floors: Carpet Stains

1/2 cup white vinegar
2 tablespoons salt

Combine ingredients until a soft paste forms. Rub paste into carpet stain and allow to dry completely. It is very important to make sure paste is completely dry and not damp. Vacuum up stain and chalky residue with a vacuum cleaner.

Floors: Carpet Stains, Heavy

1/2 cup white vinegar
2 tablespoons salt
2 tablespoons borax

Dissolve salt and borax in white vinegar. Rub solution into heavily soiled carpet stain and allow to air dry completely. After completely dry, use vacuum cleaner to vacuum up stain and any chalky residue that is left behind.

Floors: Carpet Stains, Water Stains

This is an excellent solution to remove stained carpet that has gotten wet, and left a stain from its own backing.

1/4 cup white vinegar
1 cup water

Combine vinegar and water together. Wet the stain with vinegar and water solution, and blot dry with a paper towel or clean rag. Repeat, if necessary, until water stain is gone.

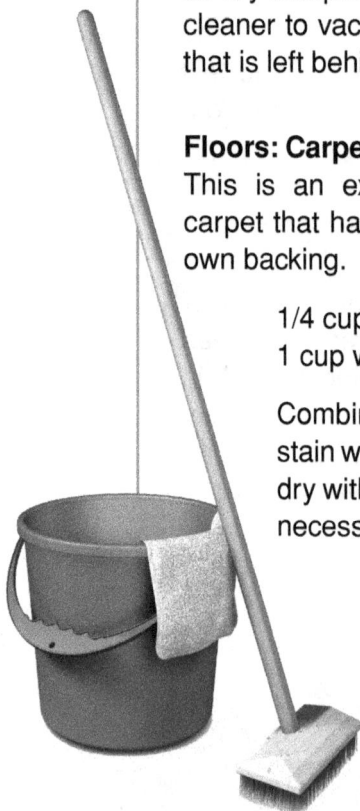

Floor Cleaner

1/2 cup white vinegar
1/4 cup liquid soap
1/4 cup lemon juice
2 gallons water

Combine all ingredients in a clean bucket. Use to wash floors that need cleaned and brightened.

Floor Cleaner, Wax Build Up

Vinegar can dissolve preexisting wax on floors. Use small amounts to achieve clean and shine. Move to higher concentration to remove wax and dirt build up.

2 cups white vinegar, divided
floor soap
bucket of water

Add 1 cup white vinegar to bucket of soapy water. Wash floor. Empty bucket and fill with water and 1 cup white vinegar. Rinse floors with vinegar water.

Furniture: Polish

1/8 cup white vinegar
1/4 cup linseed oil
1/8 cup whiskey

Combine all ingredients together in a small bowl. Use to wipe and polish furniture with a soft cloth. Allow alcohol to evaporate as solution air dries.

Furniture: Polish

3/4 cup white vinegar
1/4 cup lemon oil

Combine ingredients and store in a jar with a tight-fitting lid. Use as needed to polish furniture by wiping to a shine with a soft, clean cloth.

Furniture: Polish and Cleaner

1/2 cup white vinegar
1/2 cup olive oil

Combine both ingredients and pour into a jar with a fitted lid. Use a clean cloth or rag to wipe solution onto wood furniture and buff dry.

Flooring: Waxed Surfaces

The key to washing waxed surfaces is to use cool water instead of warm. Warm water softens the wax coating making it easier for tiny particles of dirt and dust to become embedded in the wax, dulling shine.

1/2 cup white vinegar
small bucket of cool water

Add white vinegar to bucket of cool water. Wash down waxed surfaces with a clean rag soaked in vinegar solution, or a damp mop. Dry smaller surfaces with a clean cloth, and allow wax flooring to air dry.

Furniture: Wood Cleaning

1 teaspoon white vinegar
1 cup warm water

Combine vinegar and water. Carefully wash wood surfaces to prevent haze build up common with commercial cleaners. Buff dry in a circular motion.

Furniture: Wood Paneling

1 tablespoon white vinegar
1 tablespoon olive oil
1 cup warm water

Mix all ingredients together in a small bowl. Using a clean cloth, wipe down wood paneling to perk up appearance and restore shine.

Furniture: Wood Scratches
2 tablespoons white vinegar
2 tablespoons iodine
small artist brush

Combine white vinegar and iodine together in a small dish. Using an artist's brush, paint mixture deep into scratches and allow to air dry.

For light colored scratches, add more vinegar.

For dark colored scratches, add more iodine.

Microwave
1/4 cup apple cider vinegar
1 cup water

Mix vinegar and water in a small, microwavable bowl and heat in microwave for 5 minutes. This will eliminate lingering food odors, and soften baked on food splatters making them easy to wipe off with a damp cloth.

Sharp Knives
white vinegar, undiluted
spray bottle
clay pot

Spray vinegar onto bottom of a clay pot. Sharpen knife by using clay pot as a whetstone.

Sponges
1/4 cup white vinegar
4 cups water

Rinse sponges in kitchen sink and wring out. Place water and vinegar in a bucket, and place sponges in vinegar water. Allow to soak clean overnight before wringing out.

Stainless Steel

white vinegar, undiluted
1-2 tablespoons baking soda

Dampen a cleaning cloth with vinegar and dip into baking soda to coat. Rub onto stainless steel in a circular motion. Rinse with clean water and buff with dry side of cloth until shiny clean.

Stainless Steel

white vinegar, undiluted
soft cloth

Dampen soft cloth with undiluted white vinegar. Wipe down and clean stainless steel appliances. Polish dry without rinsing.

Stainless Steel, Sinks

Use this formula to clean rust stains from stainless steel sink drains

1 tablespoon white vinegar
1 teaspoon salt

Pour salt over rust-stained spot in the sink drain. Drizzle vinegar over salt and clean with a paper towel or cleaning cloth to remove rust.

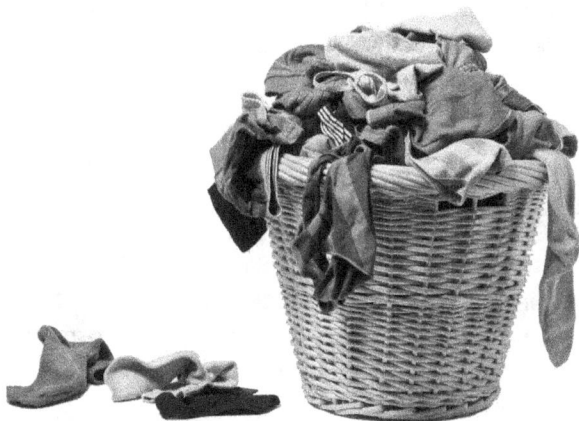

Laundry

Laundry: Alpaca Fabric
1 tablespoon white vinegar
sink basin with clean, cool water

After washing alpaca fabric as normal, rinse fabric in clean water which white vinegar has been added.

Laundry: Angora
2 tablespoons white vinegar
sink basin with clean, cool water

After normal method of washing, rinse angora in basin of clean water with white vinegar added. Gently remove excess water, without wringing, and lay flat to dry.

Laundry: Cigarette or Cigar Smoke
3 cups white vinegar
tub of very hot water

After washing clothing, hang odored clothing above bathtub. Pour vinegar into tub with very hot water, and allow steam to rid clothing of smoke. Repeat, if necessary.

Laundry: Clean and Whiten
1/2 cup white vinegar
wash load

Add undiluted white vinegar to laundry's wash cycle to clean and whiten clothes. Adding vinegar will also help kill fungus growth and inhibit mold. Run through rinse cycle as usual.

Laundry: Cotton
3/4 cup white vinegar

Add undiluted white vinegar to laundry machine's rinse cycle. Run as normal for softer cotton clothing. Great for cotton blankets and sheets, too.

Laundry: Diapers
This is a good solution for use in washing baby's cloth diapers. Vinegar will help disinfect, as well as discourage diaper rashes on baby's bottom.

3/4 cup white vinegar

Add white vinegar to final rinse water for diapers (diapers should always be rinsed twice). Fabric softeners should not be added to baby's diaper rinse water. These chemical softeners may irritate baby's delicate skin, and can make diapers less absorbing.

Laundry: Fabric Softener, Gentle
Use this for scent-free laundry. Excellent for people who are allergic to chemical softeners.

1/3 cup white vinegar

Add undiluted white vinegar to wash's final rinse cycle.

Laundry: Fabric Softener, Scent-Free
1/3 cup white vinegar
1/3 cup baking soda

Combine white vinegar and baking soda in a cup. Add to final rinse water for soft, scent-free laundry every time.

Laundry: Fabric Softener, Scented
1/2 cup apple cider vinegar
1/3 cup baking soda

Combine vinegar and baking soda in a cup. Add to final rinse water for a scented softener.

Laundry: Leather Cleaning
1/2 cup white vinegar
2-3 vitamin E capsules
1/2 cup olive oil

Bring white vinegar to boil in a small saucepan. Add vitamin E capsules and allow the capsules to dissolve completely. Remove from stovetop and add olive oil, and stir until all ingredients are well blended. Cool solution and use to clean leather coats and boots.

Laundry: Leather Polish
1/3 cup white vinegar
2/3 cup linseed oil
1/3 cup water
2 soft cloths

Combine all ingredients together in a bowl or small tub. Apply to leather with a soft cloth. Using a second, clean cloth, buff to a high shine.

Laundry: Leather Saddles and Boots
1/4 cup white vinegar
beeswax, enough to make into a cleaning paste
few drops of liquid soap
few drops of oil

Work beeswax into white vinegar which has been slightly heated on stovetop. Add soap and oil. Heat until all ingredients are soft and mixed together, then cool. Use to clean horse saddles and cowboy boots.

Laundry: Leather Shoes
1 tablespoon white vinegar
1 tablespoon rubbing alcohol
1 teaspoon vegetable oil
3-4 drops liquid soap
2 clean cloths

Combine all ingredients together in a small bowl. Using a clean cloth, gently wipe solution onto leather area of shoes. Using a second clean cloth, buff until a high shine.

Laundry: Leather Shoes, Patent
white vinegar, undiluted
1 teaspoon petroleum jelly
paper towel

Moisten a paper towel with undiluted white vinegar and gently rub into clean patent leather shoes. Using a second paper towel, finish by rubbing a slight amount of petroleum jelly into leather shoes and buff to a beautiful shine.

Laundry: Lint Trap
Hard water can cause mineral buildup on washing machine lint traps. Use this solution to occasionally clean the trap.

white vinegar, undiluted
cleaning brush

Soak lint trap in undiluted white vinegar for 2 hours. Brush away all mineral deposits clean with a cleaning brush. Rinse with clean water and replace.

For heavily built up deposits, this may need to be repeated a second time.

Laundry: Musty Smell from Bedding or Drapes
apple cider vinegar, undiluted
soft cloth or hand towel

Saturate cloth or hand towel with vinegar and wring out. Place musty bedding in clothes dryer along with vinegared cloth. Set clothes dryer setting to "Air Dry" and run for 10 to 15 minutes, allowing vinegared cloth to soak up musty odors. Repeat, if necessary, or hang outside to complete drying.

Laundry: Natural Red Dye Coloring
This solution allows you to make your very own natural red dye for fabrics.

1/2 cup vinegar
1 pound beets
1 quart water

Wash beets and place them in a saucepan; cover with cool water. Simmer beets until they become tender, then remove skins. Chop beets and return to same water in which they were cooked. Allow beets to set for 2 hours. Strain off red liquid and combine with vinegar to achieve a beautiful, natural red dye.

Laundry: Panty Hose Revitalizer
This works wonders on stretched out panty hose.

1/4 cup white vinegar
1 quart warm water

In a small bowl or clean sink basin, combine vinegar and warm water. Soak panty hose for 5 minutes. Remove and gently squeeze out excess moisture, being careful not to wring panty hose. Blot with a towel. Allow panty hose to air dry, spread out flat on a towel to help soak up excess water.

Laundry: Pretreater
1 tablespoons white vinegar
2 tablespoons ammonia
2 tablespoons baking soda
1 tablespoon liquid laundry detergent
cool water
plastic spray bottle

Pour vinegar, ammonia and liquid laundry detergent into a spray bottle. Mix together by gently swirling and add baking soda. When reactions stop foaming, add water to within an inch of the top of the bottle. Use as a pretreater for hard to clean areas and stains.

This should not be stored indefinitely in the spray bottle, as the ingredients may damage the pump.

Laundry: Removing/Adding Hems to Clothing
white vinegar, undiluted
iron

Dampen letdown hems with white vinegar prior to ironing to eliminate creases.

To add creases to fabric or hems, again dampen with vinegar and iron in a new crease.

Laundry: Remove Clothing Manufacturing Chemicals
Many people find themselves allergic to manufacturing dyes in new clothing. Use this solution to remove the chemicals prior to wearing or using for the first time.

1/4 cup white vinegar
regular wash load

Add white vinegar to laundry's wash cycle when washing new clothes for the first time. Run through cycle as usual.

Laundry: Rinse

These ready-to-go, presoaked cloths are easy to add to the final rinse cycle. They not only save measuring each time you do laundry, but keep vinegar from coming into direct contact with delicate fabrics.

white vinegar, undiluted
clean washcloths
plastic container with lid or sealing plastic bag

Soak washcloths in vinegar until saturated. Place cloths, one on top of another, in small plastic container or zipping plastic bag. Toss in one of these pretreated cloths into final rinse cycle of your washing machine.

Laundry: Saddle Soap

1/4 cup white vinegar
1/8 cup liquid soap
1/8 cup linseed oil
1/4 cup beeswax

Warm beeswax slowly over medium heat, and add vinegar. Add soap, oil, and stir together. Keep mixture warm until it blends into a smooth texture. Remove from heat and cool until it reaches a solid state.

When ready to use, rub saddle soap into leather, then buff to a high shine with a soft, clean cloth.

Laundry: Setting Fabric Dyes

Use this formula to help "set" dyes after coloring

1 cup white vinegar
1 gallon cold water
1 teaspoon salt

Fill bucket or sink with cold water. Add vinegar and salt. Soak newly dyed fabric in solution for 1 hour. Rinse in cold water to complete setting the dye.

Laundry: Silks
2 tablespoons white vinegar

Add undiluted white vinegar to final rinse cycle and run as usual. Do not rinse vinegar out.

Laundry: Stain Removal
3 tablespoons white vinegar
3 tablespoons milk

Combine ingredients together in a small bowl. Pour directly onto stain and gently rub fabric together. Allow to sit 5 minutes, then wash as usual.

Laundry: Stain Removal, Coffee and Tea Stains (dry)
This solution works best on coffee and tea stains that have already dried.

White vinegar, undiluted

Soak stain in undiluted white vinegar for 30 minutes. Wash as normal to finish removing stain. If stain does not come out completely, repeat the process again *before* drying.

Laundry: Stain Removal, Coffee and Tea Stains (wet)
This solution works best on wet coffee and tea stains.

white vinegar, undiluted
clean water
liquid laundry detergent

Blot out as much coffee or tea as possible with a paper towel. Rinse in cool water, and wring out slightly. Pour white vinegar directly onto stain. Wash in lukewarm, soapy water.

Laundry: Stain Removal, Coffee and Tea Stains (stubborn)

Try this solution to remove stubborn stain.

White vinegar, undiluted
1 teaspoon salt

Wet stained area with vinegar. Sprinkle damped stain with salt and set garment in bright sunlight for at least one hour. Wash and dry garment as usual. For tough stains, you may need to repeat this process.

Laundry: Stain Removal, Ink

1 tablespoon white vinegar
1 tablespoon cornstarch
milk, enough to cover stain

Soak ink stain in milk for one hour. Combine white vinegar and cornstarch into a paste. Cover the stain with paste and gently rub into cloth. Leave stain until paste dries, then wash as usual.

Laundry: Stain Removal, Iron Scorching

white vinegar, undiluted
1 teaspoon salt
clean cloth

Dampen a clean cloth with white vinegar. Blot vinegar onto scorched area and allow to set for 5 minutes. If stain remains, repeat. If after 2 attempts scorching still remains, sprinkle salt over remoistened scorch and allow to set for 5 minutes. Wash as usual.

Laundry: Stain Removal, Permanent Press

white vinegar, undiluted

Wet stain with white vinegar, and allow to set for 3 to 5 minutes. Wash in cool water and rinse clean.

Laundry: Stain Removal, Perspiration Stains
1/4 cup white vinegar
2 gallons water

Combine white vinegar and water in a clean sink. Soak perspiration stained clothing in solution overnight. Wash as usual.

Laundry: Stain Removal, Rust Stains
1 tablespoon white vinegar
1 teaspoon salt

Pour vinegar directly over rust stain, making sure to use enough vinegar to cover stain entirely. Sprinkle salt over dampened stain. Set outside in the sun for at least an hour to dry. Rinse out salt and reapply until stain disappears completely. Wash as usual.

Laundry: Stain Removal, Wine
This is a strong formula for removing tough wine stains. Be careful to work gently into delicate fabrics.

1 tablespoon white vinegar
3 tablespoons water
1 teaspoon salt

Blot up as much wine as possible from fabric. Saturate stain with white vinegar and water. While stain is still wet with vinegar solution, gently rub salt into stain. Set in sunlight to dry completely, then wash as usual.

Laundry: Stain Removal, Wine
white vinegar, undiluted

Blot undiluted white vinegar onto a wine stain. Stain will begin to dissipate and fade immediately. Wash as usual.

Laundry: Static Cling
1/4 cup white vinegar
rinse load

Add white vinegar to laundry's final rinse cycle to eliminate static cling and reduce lint.

Laundry: Straw Hats
Straw hats can become worn out and misshapen over time. Try this formula to bring new life to an old straw hat.

1 teaspoon white vinegar
1/2 cup salt
bucket of water plus 1 cup water
few drops liquid detergent, if necessary
spray bottle.

Put salt in a bucket of warm water and dissolve completely. Submerge straw hat in salt water solution. Once straw is slightly softened, remove from salt water and wipe away any stains. For tough stains, add a drop or two of liquid detergent to a sponge and wipe clean. Push and mold straw hat back into original shape.

Put vinegar and 1 cup of water in a spray bottle. Once hat is in desired shape, spray hat with a fine mist of vinegar solution. Allow to air dry, but do not dry in direct sunlight.

Laundry: Wool Sweaters
1 cup white vinegar

Add vinegar to laundry machine's rinse cycle and run as normal. Wool sweaters will come out fluffy after vinegar rinse.

Baby Bottle Nipples
1 teaspoon white vinegar
2 cups water

In a clean pan, add vinegar and water together and drop in baby bottle nipples. Bring to a boil and continue boiling for several minutes. This will not only clean and sterilize nipples, but also keep them from developing a sour taste.

High Chair Cleaning
white vinegar, undiluted
spray bottle
cleaning cloth

Set high chair in the shower and spray with full strength vinegar. Allow to set for 5-10 minutes. Turn shower on with warm water and spray high chair for 3 minutes. Wipe food and grime off chair. Give a final rinse and wipe dry.

Odors
This is a great, non-invasive method for eliminating odor from baby's nursery.

White vinegar, undiluted
spray bottle
damp towel taken from washing machine

Take a clean towel that has just been washed, but still damp, form the washing machine. Spray damp towel with vinegar and hang over door in baby's room. As towel dries it will work to control odors and add clean moisture to the room.

Play Clay for Children

Here is a fun, non-toxic recipe for play clay that is completely natural and safe for children to use.

1 teaspoon white vinegar
1 cup flour
1/2 cup salt
1 cup water
1 tablespoon oil
food coloring, if desired

Combine all ingredients in a saucepan over medium heat. Stir continually until it forms into a ball. Remove from heat and allow to cool. Knead clay ball until smooth. Add a few drops of food coloring, if desired. Store in a tightly sealed container or wrapped in plastic wrap in the refrigerator.

Toys

1/4 white vinegar
1 cup water

In a small bowl, combine vinegar and water. Use this solution to wipe down baby toys, plastic dolls, and building blocks.

Toys

1/4 cup white vinegar
1 quart hot water
few drops of dish detergent

Combine all ingredients in a bowl or small tub. Use to wash down baby toys. Rinse well and dry.

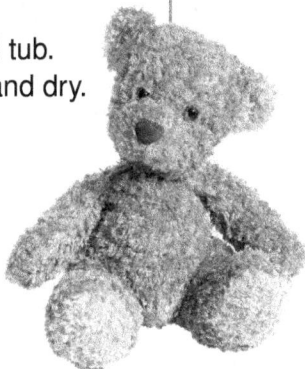

Books
1 tablespoon white vinegar
2 cups water
spray bottle

Using a fine mist spray bottle, spray a soft cloth with this weak vinegar solution. Use cloth to wipe books and dry immediately.

Bookshelves
2 cups white vinegar
bucket of warm water
few drops of liquid detergent

Add vinegar, water and a few drops of liquid detergent to bucket. Using a rag or sponge, wipe down bookshelves, being certain to get into corners and crevices.

Construction Paper Stains
Colored construction paper, when it becomes wet, can leaved colored stains on desks and other furniture. Try this formula for simple and thorough removal.

1/4 cup white vinegar
1/4 cup water

Combine both vinegar and water together. Use paper towels to blot up wet construction paper stains.

Correction Fluid
white vinegar, undiluted

Dab area of furniture or cushion that has unwanted

correction fluid. Gently wipe with a paper towel to clean. If spot is persistent, slightly saturate stain with vinegar and blot away.

Super Glue on Fingers
white vinegar, undiluted
small bowl

Fill a small bowl with undiluted white vinegar. Soak affected fingers for several minutes. Peel away stuck glue.

Around the House

Air Freshener
1 tablespoon white vinegar
1 teaspoon baking soda
2 cups water
spray bottle

Combine ingredients in a plastic spray bottle. Spray into the air in rooms needing a freshening up.

All-Purpose Cleaner
This is a great, all-purpose cleaning solution to have on hand for many cleaning jobs around the house.

1/4 cup white vinegar
2 cups water
3 tablespoons liquid detergent
plastic spray bottle.

Combine all ingredients in a plastic spray bottle. Use around the house for every day household cleaning. It is a great cleaner for high dust areas, like banisters and window baseboards, too.

Ceilings

1/2 cup white vinegar
1 tablespoon dish detergent
half bucket of warm water

Combine all ingredients in a bucket. In sections, use sponge or cloth to wash. Dry each section before you begin a new one. A new paint roller brush on an extended broom handle works well for this, too.

Room Deodorizer

1 cup apple cider vinegar
1/4 cup water
1 tablespoon cinnamon

Heat vinegar and water on stovetop until hot. Remove from heat and pour into a bowl. Sprinkle cinnamon on top of vinegar solution. Place bowl on a low table in room to be freshened.

Painted Surfaces

1/4 cup white vinegar
1 tablespoon cornstarch
2 cups hot water

Combine ingredients in a bowl or storage cup. Wipe or spray solution onto painted surface. Immediately dry with a cloth. Do not allow liquid to soak into paint.

Painting: Concrete Walls and Floors

This solution will help prepare concrete walls and floors for painting, cutting down on future peeling.

White vinegar, undiluted
brush or roller

Brush or paint concrete walls or floors with undiluted white vinegar as a preparation for painting. Allow to air dry thoroughly before applying paint.

Painting: Odor-Free Painting
3 cups white vinegar or apple cider vinegar

Fill 3 small bowls with 1 cup vinegar in each bowl. Place around room being painted to help absorb fresh paint odors while painting.

Painting: Remove Old Paint from Wood Windows
1/2 cup white vinegar
1/2 cup liquid detergent
paintbrush
razor blade or scraper

Combine vinegar and liquid detergent and mix. Use a paintbrush to brush vinegar mixture onto wood that needs paint to be removed. Soak for 10 minutes, then begin to carefully scrape away old paint with a razor scraper.

Walls
2 cups white vinegar, divided
bucket of warm water
few drops of dish detergent

Combine all ingredients in a bucket. Using a clean rag, wipe walls and allow to air dry. For markings on wall that do not seem to wipe away, try a quick rub with undiluted vinegar. Fill bucket with warm rinse water. Add another cup of vinegar. Use this solution with a clean cloth to rinse walls clean.

Wallpaper Stripping
1 cup white vinegar
1 tablespoon liquid detergent
spray bottle

Combine vinegar and detergent in a spray bottle. Wet wallpaper surface with vinegar solution and allow to set for 5 minutes. Gently remove wallpaper with scraper, adding more solution as you go. For difficult jobs, try "etching" wallpaper first with a scoring tool. Then wet wallpaper with solution and allow to set for another 5 minutes. Wallpaper should now peel or scrape free.

Window Cleaner, Streak Free
1/4 cup white vinegar
1 quart water
spray bottle

Combine all ingredients in a plastic spray bottle. Spray onto windows and mirrors. Wipe immediately with a soft cloth or paper towel.

Window Cleaner, Deep Cleaning
1/4 cup white vinegar
1/4 cup cornstarch

Combine ingredients together and dab thick solution onto dirty windows. Allow to dry to a chalky film. Rub off with a soft cloth in a circular motion until clean.

Window Cleaner, Cleaning Cloths
1/4 cup white vinegar
1/2 teaspoon liquid dish soap
2 cups water

Combine all ingredients together in a bowl. Using a clean cloth, dip into mixture and wring out. Store damp coated cloth in a glass jar with tight fitting lid. Wipe spots from windows and mirrors, as needed.

Windows: Drapes

This is a wonderful solution to freshen up drapery from existing odors and add a new freshness to the room. Be sure your drapes are free of heavy dust before wetting. Dust can be eliminated with tools from your vacuum cleaner.

1 tablespoon white vinegar
2 cups warm water
spray bottle

In a plastic bottle, combine warm water and vinegar, and shake gently to combine. Spritz each drapery panel and moisten drapes, paying particular attention to add a little extra solution to any heavily wrinkled areas.

Allow to air dry, still hanging on the windows. Drapes will smell fresher, and most of all, the wrinkles will disappear.

Windows: Drapes, Fiberglass

Fiberglass drapes demand special attention when getting cleaned. Try this formula to clean fiberglass drapes, while still keeping their delicate integrity.

1 tablespoon white vinegar
2 cups water
plastic spray bottle
garden hose
outdoor clothesline

Hang drapes firmly on a clothesline and spray gently with a hose, fully wetting the drapes. Fill plastic spray bottle with water and vinegar. Spray drapes with vinegar solution and allow to dry on clothesline for ultimate freshness.

Windows: Shutters and Louvered Doors
white vinegar, undiluted
spray bottle
paint stirring stick or ruler
soft clean cloth

Fill a spray bottle with undiluted vinegar. Wrap a soft clean cloth around a paint stirring stick or ruler. Spray cloth with vinegar and run it over and beneath each louver to get rid of dust.

Miscellaneous

Ash Trays
1/8 cup white vinegar
1/8 cup hot water

Combine white vinegar and hot water. Fill ashtray and allow to sit overnight to get rid of lingering smoke odors.

Aquariums
This solution is excellent for cleaning the outside glass of a fish aquarium. However, it should *never* be used to clean the inside, as the vinegar could be toxic to fish. Always spray vinegar onto cloth, and not directly on aquarium glass. Tiny droplets may get into the aquarium water and upset the delicate pH balance, possibly harming fish.

1 teaspoon white vinegar
1 cup water
spray bottle
clean cloth

Combine the white vinegar and water and pour into a spray bottle. Spray soft cloth with vinegar solution and wipe clean aquarium exterior. Buff dry. If aquarium exterior is extremely dirty, use undiluted vinegar and wipe clean.

Ballpoint Pen Stains
white vinegar, undiluted
clean cloth

Wet area stained with ballpoint pen with vinegar. You can do this by drizzling vinegar over the area and allow to penetrate the stained area of cloth. For areas that are vertical, like walls, soak a clean cloth in vinegar and place against stain. Allow to soak in for 10 minutes. Blot up with a clean cloth. Repeat, if necessary. Thoroughly dry, when finished.

Chewing Gum
white vinegar, undiluted

Soak chewing gum in undiluted vinegar. Soak until chewing gum begins to dissolve. If chewing gum will not dissolve, repeat above steps with heated vinegar.

Eyeglasses
1 tablespoon white vinegar
cotton ball or soft cloth

Drench cotton ball or soft cloth with white vinegar. Wipe eyeglasses clean and allow to air dry, streak free.

Fireplace Ashes

This vinegar water solution keeps ashes from flying around the room and helps neutralize alkali in the ash.

2 tablespoons white vinegar
2 cups water
spray bottle

Fill spray bottle with vinegar and water. Before scooping out ashes, spray them down with a coating of vinegar and water solution. Now scoop out wet ashes (this will help keep them from flying all over the room). Continue to spray as you clean to keep dust and ash particles to a minimum. When finished scooping out ashes, use remaining vinegar solution to thoroughly clean fireplace if finished using for the season.

Garbage Cans

1 cup white vinegar
1/2 gallon water

Pour a half gallon of water in an empty garbage can and add vinegar. Swirl around bottom and edges of can and then place in direct sunlight. As it dries, it will not only disinfect, but also rid can of lingering garbage odors.

Glass or Beaded Jewelry

1 tablespoon white vinegar
2 quarts warm water, divided
1 teaspoon liquid detergent

Combine 1 quart of water and liquid detergent. Dip strand of beads into water. Remove immediately and dip into second bowl of warm water and vinegar to rinse clean. Blot dry with a paper towel and complete drying with hair dryer on lowest setting.

Hairbrushes
1/2 cup white vinegar
2 cups hot water
2-3 drops liquid dish soap

Combine vinegar, hot water and a few drops of liquid soap. Completely immerse hairbrushes in vinegar solution and allow to soak for 30 minutes. Rub hairbrushes together to clean and rinse thoroughly. Allow to air dry.

Hairbrushes, Combs and Rollers
1 cup white vinegar, plus 1/4 cup white vinegar
1 quart warm water, plus extra water
few drops liquid dish detergent
old toothbrush

Combine 1 cup white vinegar and warm water in a large bowl or sink. Place brushes, combs and rollers in vinegar water and allow to soak for one hour. Remove and brush away any lingering build up with old toothbrush to which a few drops of liquid detergent has been added. Rinse with clear water.

Refill sink basin with warm water and add 1/4 cup more white vinegar. Rinse brushes and combs clean one last time. Allow to air dry on a towel.

Humidifiers
2 tablespoons white vinegar
humidifier water

Add two tablespoons of white vinegar to water in a humidifier to eliminate odors in your home as it humidifies. Vinegar also discourages bacteria and mold growth in the humidifier's water receptacle.

Lamp Shades

2 cups white vinegar, undiluted
3 tablespoons liquid detergent
bucket or small tub of hot water

Combine white vinegar and liquid detergent in bucket of hot water. Take and old lamp shade and immerse one corner of shade in tub of water, and move it around vigorously to clean. Take shade out, turn to a different corner, and repeat until entire shade has been cleaned. Remove shade from water and empty tub. Refill tub with clean water and add another cup of vinegar. Repeat same clean and shake motion to now rinse lampshade. Allow to air dry.

Moth Repellent

1/2 cup white vinegar
1/4 cup lavender
small cloth or sachet

Combine white vinegar and lavender in a small jar. Leave jar open in moth-ridden areas.

Also saturate small cloths or sachets with this solution, and place in areas you wish to rid of moths.

Moth Repellent

2 cups white vinegar
1/2 cup lavender leaves

Heat vinegar over stovetop and add torn lavender leaves. Simmer for 10 minutes and remove from heat. Allow to cool completely.

Pour into jar with a tight-fitting lid. Allow to steep for 10 days. Use to wipe down walls and plastic storage bins in clothes closet to drive away moths.

Silk House Plants
1/4 cup white vinegar
1 quart water

Combine both ingredients in a small bowl. Use paper towel or cleaning rag to dab in solution and wipe dust and dirt from silk and plastic house plants. Allow to air dry. You can also pour this solution into a plastic spray bottle and use to spray silk plants to keep dust from forming in the first place.

Sticker or Decal Removal
white vinegar, undiluted
cotton ball or paper towel

Wet a cotton ball or paper towel with vinegar and saturate sticker or decal. Soak until sticker or decal can be removed. Repeat if necessary until sticker and glue residue comes free.

For stickers or decals that will not come free, gently scratch the top layer off, or scratch grooves into the paper. Then, repeat steps above, allowing to soak until sticker breaks free.

Urine Stained Mattress
This solution will not only remove unsightly urine stains from mattresses, but also the unpleasant odor that accompanies it.

white vinegar, undiluted
spray bottle
soft cloths or paper towels

Spray urine stained area of mattress with undiluted vinegar, and allow to set for 2-3 minutes. Use a cloth or paper towel to blot dry. May need to repeat process until entire stain comes clean.

Wet Dry Vac

Wet Dry Vacs tend to smell musty after time. Try using this formula periodically to freshen vac and extend the life of this appliance.

1 cup white vinegar
1 quart warm water

Combine vinegar and warm water together. Suck up solution in vac and set for 5 minutes. Empty machine and wipe out inside of vac. Allow vac to air dry completely before putting it back together for storage.

Septic System

1/2 cup white vinegar
1/2 cup baking soda
hot water
1 package dry yeast
2/3 cup brown sugar

First, clean drains throughout the house by pouring baking soda down drain, and follow with white vinegar. Allow each drain to rest with baking soda and vinegar solution for 10 minutes. Then, run hot water down drain to rinse clean.

Next, pour yeast and brown sugar into toilet and flush tank twice.

Schedule this preventative maintenance by putting it on your calendar! Doing this routine monthly will not only keep drains running clean, but also help septic system to run efficiently for many years.

Chapter Six

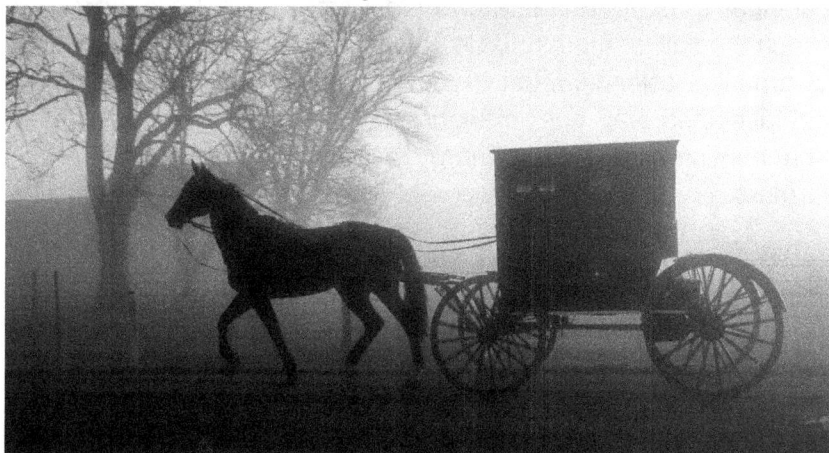

Amish Farming & More

Nobody does farming better than the Amish. A simple drive by an Amish farm or community is an idyllic vision of golden crops ready for harvest by horse-drawn plows and orchards brimming with lush fruits. These wonderful people are known for their farming skills above all else. People drive for miles to purchase a portion of the leftover crop at Amish produce stands, knowing they are buying quality fresh foods, rich in flavor and picked at the peak of freshness.

Amish farms are the picture of abundance.

As a general rule, most Amish farmers do so foremost to provide for their families. Then, the excess bounty which their families cannot use is sold at roadside stands, farmers' markets or Amish stores.

Farming and gardening skills are passed down through the family line. They are experts in crop rotation, and many Amish farms avoid the use of dangerous chemical pesticides opting for more natural farming solutions.

While the Amish are often referred to as a 'plain people,' they are far from simple. Instead of using a predetermined date on the calendar to plant, rotate and harvest crops, they have learned to watch the soil for more reliable clues. They have a deep knowledge of practical science when it comes to farming. And, farming the old-fashioned way has allowed Amish farmers to produce more abundant crops using less energy resources than that of non-Amish farmers.

There is much we can learn from watching how Amish farms are sown, cared for and cultivated. By getting back to basics we can avoid costly mistakes and reap a bountiful harvest on the time and money we have invested.

Cut Flowers
1 tablespoon white vinegar
2 cups water
2 tablespoons sugar

Combine all ingredients in a vase and add cut flowers with stems cut at an angle for beautiful, long-lasting blooms.

Birdbaths
This solution is great for controlling growth of fungus and bacteria in outdoor bird baths.

2 tablespoons white vinegar

Add white vinegar to outdoor birdbath water every time you refill the bird bath to keep water bacteria free, and fresh for drinking.

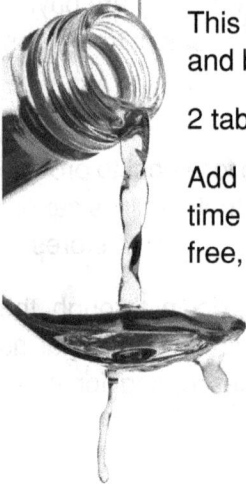

Fruit Flies
1 cup apple cider vinegar
few drops liquid dish detergent
glass jar (mason size)
plastic wrap
rubber band
toothpick

Pour a cup of apple cider vinegar into a glass mason jar and add a few drops of liquid detergent. Poke a few tiny holes in the plastic wrap with a toothpick and place over mouth of glass jar. Secure in place with a rubber band and place on kitchen counter near fruit.

Fruit flies will be attracted to the apple cider vinegar and fall into the liquid. The liquid detergent acts as a barrier in the water and fruit flies will be unable to get back out.

Hummingbird Feeders
white vinegar, undiluted

Use white vinegar to clean and disinfect and empty hummingbird feeder. Rinse and wipe dry before using.

Soaps and detergents can be toxic to delicate birds, but because vinegar is natural, it makes the perfect cleaning solution that is powerful enough to disinfect, but delicate enough not to harm birds.

Outdoor Water Fountains
1/2 - 1 cup white vinegar

Add white vinegar to outdoor water fountains to keep fountain pumps running clean, disinfect from bacteria and discourage mold or moss growth.

Rusty Tools
white vinegar, undiluted

Using liberal amounts of white vinegar, wash down rusty garden tools allowing the rusted areas to become completely soaked in vinegar. Allow to set for 10 minutes and wipe away rust.

Cats in Sandbox
white vinegar

Sprinkle white vinegar in a child's sandbox to prevent roaming cats from using the box as their personal litter box.

Garden Problems: Balance Soil pH Level
1 cup white vinegar
bucket of water

Pour white vinegar into bucket of clean water. Pour in a circle around acid-loving plants, such as azaleas, blueberries, marigolds and radishes to balance soil's pH level.

Garden Problems: Clay Flowerpots
white vinegar, undiluted
scrub brush
clean water

Mineral deposits not only make the pots appear unsightly, but can also interfere with the way clay pots breathe and absorb water.

Dip scrub brush in white vinegar and scrub the outside of pots. If pot is empty, also clean the inside of the pot. Use fresh water to rinse pot clean.

Garden Problems: Cucumber and Melon Plants
2 cups white vinegar
1/4 cup oregano leaves

Combine vinegar and oregano together and allow to set for at least 15 minutes. Wet ground area around cucumber or melon plants every week to keep bugs from eating plants.

Garden Problems: Fungus
1 tablespoon vinegar
1 cup chamomile tea

Combine vinegar and chamomile tea and spray onto plants to safely eliminate fungus.

Garden Problems: Herbicide
Try this mixture on hard-to-kill vegetation infiltrating gardens and walk paths. It can also be used to kill any unwanted grass growing in the cracks of driveways or sidewalks.

2 quarts white vinegar
1/3 cup salt
1 tablespoon liquid dish detergent
1 teaspoon cayenne pepper
spray bottle

Combine white vinegar and salt in a bowl and stir until salt is completely dissolved. Pour vinegar salt mixture in plastic spray bottle and add liquid dish detergent and cayenne pepper.

Use this solution in any vegetation you want to kill, paying particular attention to completely soaking the plant's leaves.

Garden Problems: Herbicide
2 cups white vinegar
1/4 cup salt
spray bottle

Combine ingredients in a spray bottle making sure to completely dissolve salt before attempting to use sprayer. Spray solution on unwanted grass or weed areas and allow to completely saturate.

Garden Problems: Insects
1/4 cup white vinegar
3/4 cup water
few drops liquid detergent
spray bottle

Combine white vinegar, water and a few drops of liquid detergent in a spray bottle. Use to spray tender garden plants that are being overtaken by troublesome insects.

Garden Problems: Nasturtiums
1/8 teaspoon white vinegar
2 cups water
nasturtium seeds

Combine white vinegar and water in a bowl and soak nasturtium seeds overnight before planting. The following morning, be sure and plant seeds while they are still damp for best and quickest growth.

Garden Problems: Okra
1/8 teaspoon white vinegar
1 1/2 cups water
okra seeds

Mix white vinegar and water in a bowl and soak okra seeds overnight before planting.

Garden Problems: Paths and Stones

1/2 cup white vinegar
1 tablespoon fresh thyme

Combine ingredients together. Sprinkle or spray onto garden paths and stepping stones as a wonderful pest repellent. This concoction will also help keep mold and mildew from forming on stones.

Garden Problems: Tomatoes
1 cup white vinegar
1/4 cup basil leaves

Combine white vinegar and chopped basil leaves and allow to set for at least 15 minutes. Soak ground beneath tomato plants to keep insects away.

Garden Problems: Varmints
white vinegar, undiluted
old rags or cloths (discarded socks can also work well for this)

Soak rags in white vinegar and place around garden as a deterrent for varmints.

Garden Problems: Varmints
apple cider vinegar
cotton balls

Soak cotton balls in apple cider vinegar and place strategically around garden. The vinegar will not only keep varmints and insects at bay, but is also helpful for balancing pH levels in soil itself.

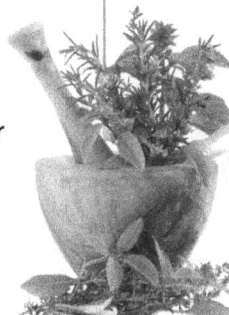

Garden Problems: Vegetables
2 cups white vinegar
1/4 cup sage, chopped

Combine white vinegar and sage together and store in a plastic bottle. Sprinkle sage vinegar around vegetable vines to keep plant-eating insects away.

Insects: Ants
white vinegar, undiluted
spray bottle

Fill a spray bottle with undiluted vinegar. Use to spray cupboards and countertops to rid home of ants.

Insects: Ants
white vinegar, undiluted
spray bottle

Pour white vinegar into a spray bottle and use to spray a defining barrier around home's entry points, such as windows and doors.

Insects: Anthills
white vinegar, undiluted

Pour undiluted white vinegar directly down anthill opening to kill the hill.

Insects: Aphids
2 cups white vinegar
1 cup mint leaves, shredded

Combine vinegar and shredded mint leaves and allow to set for 10 minutes. Wet a circle of ground around cabbage, brussels sprouts and cauliflower plants with this mint vinegar mixture to keep aphids from dining on plants.

Insects: Fire Ant Hills
white vinegar, undiluted

Saturate ant hills with undiluted vinegar to get rid of fire ants. May need to repeat, making sure vinegar is working its way down into the ant hill.

Insects: Fleas
2 cups white vinegar
1/2 cup basil, torn

Combine white vinegar and torn basil leaves together and warm on the stovetop. Simmer for 20 minutes and then cool completely. Pour in a thick line along home's entry doorways to prevent fleas from entering the house.

Insects: Flying Insects
1/4 cup white vinegar
2 bay leaves, crushed
spray bottle

Pour vinegar into plastic spray bottle. Crush bay leaves and add to vinegar. Spray down picnic table and outlying area to keep flies and other insects at bay.

Insects: Mosquitoes
2 cups white vinegar
1/2 cup lavender flowers

Warm vinegar on stovetop and add lavender flowers. Simmer for 10 minutes. Cool completely and pour into a bowl or jar. Sprinkle around yard to keep mosquitoes at bay.

Insects: Snails and Slugs
1/2 cup white vinegar
1/2 cup water
spray bottle

Combine white vinegar and water in a spray bottle and use directly on snails and slugs for elimination.

LIVESTOCK

Apple cider vinegar has proven to be an effective addition to the diet of livestock. Because apple cider vinegar is primarily acetic acid, it can be easily absorbed directly into the digestive tract of farm animals. Vinegar can help prevent an array of digestive issues in livestock, including gas, reflux, poor digestion and even internal parasitic infections. Probiotics, which are so much the current rave in farming, are naturally occurring in apple cider vinegar providing essential vitamins, minerals and nutrients. It has also been linked to the prevention and cure of ketosis.

From the standpoint of meat quality, apple cider vinegar can help improve both the flavor and texture of meats without the use of artificial chemical and dangerous additives. It is not only cost effective, but you will find that most animals enjoy the flavorful addition of apple cider vinegar to their daily diets.

Consider adding apple cider vinegar to livestock diet by:

• Adding directly to drinking water trough

• Offering an occasional special treat of a half apple cider vinegar, half water solution in a trough or bowl of its own

• Sprinkling directly onto hay or other feed for consumption.

Livestock: Cattle
apple cider vinegar

Add 2 tablespoons per gallon of water to troughs to help protect cattle and other livestock from illness.

Livestock: Chickens
1/4 teaspoon white vinegar

Add white vinegar to chickens' water each day to help support better growth. It is also thought that chickens consuming vinegar tend to be more tender, and increases egg laying.

Livestock: Chickens
white vinegar, undiluted
spray bottle

Fill a plastic spray bottle with white vinegar and use to clean and disinfect chicken coups.

Livestock: Flies
1 cup white vinegar
1 cup

Pour white vinegar and water into a spray bottle and use to spray livestock to keep irritation flies away.

Livestock: Horses
1/2 cup vinegar

Use vinegar to sprinkle directly on hay to prevent kidney stones and colic in horses.

Livestock: Pigs
1 cup apple cider vinegar

Add a cup of apple cider vinegar to a 20 gallon water tough.

Livestock: Skin Conditions
2 quarts apple cider vinegar
2 cups warm water

Combine vinegar and water and pour solution over livestock with skin rashes and itches. Allow the solution to soak into affected area and air dry. The strong vinegar smell will evaporate as the vinegar itself dries.

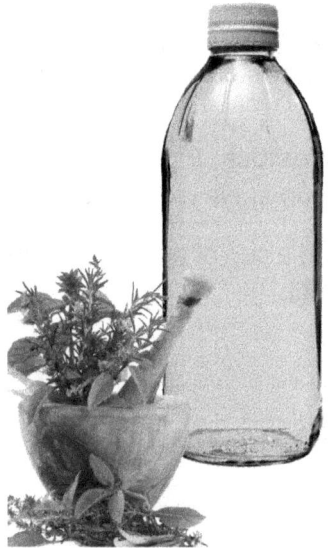

Chapter Seven

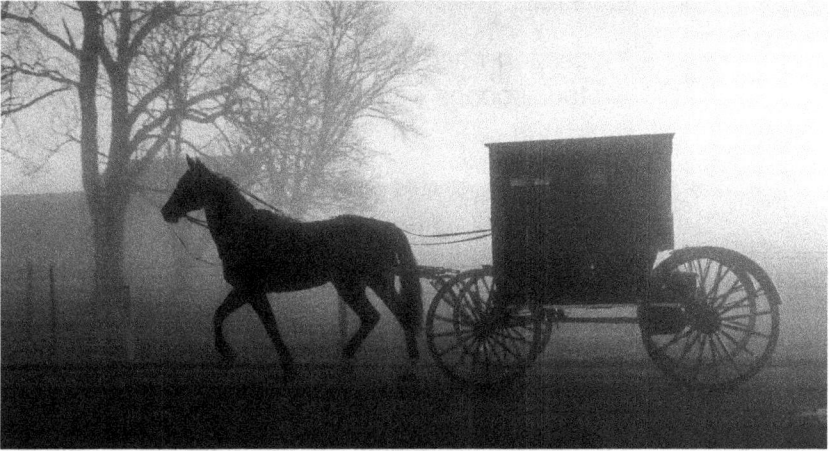

In & Around

While it comes as no surprise that vinegar is the basis for hundreds of natural healing remedies and is unparalleled in its disinfecting ability, some of its less talked about uses cannot be overlooked.

As the Amish already know, vinegar is excellent for removing invasive vegetation as well as balancing delicate pH levels in farming or gardening soil. It is highly acidic in nature and, due to its chemical makeup, possesses an innate ability to neutralize even the most foul odors.

Those same attributes make vinegar a potent degreaser and even tool revitalizer. It is not only safe for humans, but also valuable livestock and cherished pets. Its uses are nearly limitless.

The pages that follow are just a sampling of some of the less familiar, but equally useful, ways that simple vinegar can be used to better the circles we live in.

Pets: Behavior Issues

This is an easy solution to help with pet's behavior issues.

1 teaspoon white vinegar or apple cider vinegar
few tablespoons water
squirt gun

Fill squirt gun with water, leaving a small amount of room. Add white vinegar. When pet approaches a forbidden area or begins to engage in unwanted behavior (such as scratching or chewing), tell them a stern "No" and reinforce the words with a quick liquid reminder. Soon, simply picking up the squirt gun will ensure good behavior, and eventually once the bad habit is broken, no reminder will be needed at all.

Pets: Dishes

Use this vinegar solution to clean and disinfect pets' food and water dishes. Because these surfaces remain damp throughout the day, they likely harbor harmful bacteria and mold that can be unhealthy for both pets and people. Using vinegar on pets' surfaces avoids the need to use harsher chemicals, such as chlorine-based bleach, that might be harmful to the animal.

1/4 cup white vinegar
water

Pour white vinegar into pet's food or water dish and fill with water. Allow to soak for 20 minutes once a week to clean and disinfect.

Pets: Dog Itching

1/3 cup apple cider vinegar
2 quarts warm water

Shampoo and rinse dog as usual. Combine apple cider vinegar and warm water in a clean bucket and pour over dog as his final rinse. Do not rinse again. Dry dog as usual and coat will be shiny and soft, cutting down on itching and scratching.

Pets: Fleas

1 cup white vinegar
1 tablespoon rue, chopped

Combine vinegar and rue in a small bowl. Rub this concentration into dog's hair to discourage or get rid of nasty fleas.

Pets: Fleas

1/2 cup white vinegar
1/4 cup water
1 tablespoon fennel

Combine all ingredients and pour into a spray bottle. Thoroughly saturate areas where pets sleep or play with vinegar solution. Allow to air dry.

Pets: Fur

1 teaspoon apple cider vinegar

Add a teaspoon of apple cider vinegar to dog or cat's water dish to give pets a shiny, healthy coat.

Pets: Jellyfish Stings
Keep this solution on hand when taking your dog on vacation to the ocean where jellyfish may be a problem.

white vinegar or apple cider vinegar

At first suspicion of jellyfish sting, pour undiluted vinegar over sting area to help dilute the poison.

Pets: Hair
Try this easy method of removing pet hair from carpet, furniture or clothing.

white vinegar, undiluted
spray bottle
discarded sock

Turn an old tube sock inside out and slip it over your hand. Spray lightly with white vinegar and use dampened sock to wipe down furniture, carpet or clothing to remove pet hair. Dampened sock can also be used to wipe down pet directly, removing shedding hair.

Pets: Horse's Coat
1/8 cup apple cider vinegar

Pour apple cider vinegar into horse's water trough every day to help keep his coat shiny and healthy.

Pets: Illness
1 teaspoon apple cider vinegar

Add a teaspoonful of apple cider vinegar to pets' water dish to help boost immune system during an illness.

Pets: Long-Haired Cats
3 tablespoons white vinegar
1 quart water

Combine together white vinegar and warm water. After bathing cat, rinse long fur in this warm vinegar solution. Fur will shine and mats will brush out easier.

Pets: Odor
Keep a bottle full of this mixture on hand for daily odor control for all types of furry pets.

2 tablespoons white vinegar
2 cups water
spray bottle

Pour white vinegar and water into a large spray bottle. Spray pet's coat daily to help eliminate odor.

Pets: Skunk Spray
white vinegar
clean towel

Wet a clean towel with white vinegar and use to rub down a dog or cat that has been sprayed with skunk spray.

Pets: Ticks
Try using this solution before heading outdoors to protect your hunting dog from ticks.

white vinegar, undiluted
1/2 cup chamomile flowers

Combine vinegar and chamomile flowers in a small bowl. Set for 15 minutes to allow flower to thoroughly incorporate into vinegar. Wipe this mixture onto dog's coat to discourage ticks.

Pets: Urine

white vinegar, undiluted
1 tablespoon baking soda
spray bottle
scrub brush

If urine stains on carpet or flooring are still damp, blot up as much as possible with a paper towel. Using vinegar in a spray bottle, completely dampen area of urine stain. Sprinkle baking soda over dampened stain. Using a scrub brush, brush stained area in a circular motion. Allow to dry completely. When dry, vacuum up stain and residue.

It is important to be sure area is completely dry before vacuuming. Vacuuming damp residue can clog vacuum cleaner.

Pets: Urine

white vinegar, undiluted
spray bottle
paper towels

Blot up any excess urine with paper towels. Spray white vinegar directly over entire area that has been affected. Allow to soak for 2 to 3 minutes and blot up vinegar liquid with another paper towel. Repeat again, as necessary.

Air Conditioner Grills

white vinegar, undiluted
clean cloths

Using a dry cloth, wipe away any loose dirt and debris from air conditioner grills as usual. Take a second clean cloth or rag and soak with white vinegar. Use once again on air conditioner grills to remove any leftover dirt and to inhibit future dirt and dust buildup.

Barbecue Grills

2 cups white vinegar
2 tablespoons dishwasher detergent
2 quarts hot water
plastic garbage bag
spray bottle
cleaning rag

Remove soiled barbecue rack from grill and place in plastic garbage bag. Fill spray bottle with vinegar and use to spray down entire rack until wet. Tie garbage bag in a loose knot to seal in the moisture. Place bag with rack in warm sun and leave for about 4 hours.

Untie bag (be careful not to rip) and add dishwasher detergent and hot water. Retie bag and leave rack to soak in sun for an additional 2 hours. Open bag and use cleaning rag to wipe rack clean.

Boats: Stains and Discoloration

Aluminum boats are extremely sensitive to alkaline in the water, which can etch aluminum and cause discoloration. White vinegar is an excellent source to neutralize alkaline, making it easier to scrub away discoloration.

white vinegar, undiluted
clean water rinse
towel

Using a towel saturated in white vinegar, wipe clean any stains or discoloration appearing on boat. Rinse clean with clear water and wipe dry.

Campers and RVs: Fiberglass
white vinegar, undiluted
spray bottle
rinse water
paper towel

Spray areas of fiberglass camper or RV with undiluted vinegar where hard water has left stains. Wipe down with cloth and dry completely.

For tough to clean stains, soak a paper towel in vinegar and "stick" on top of stain for 5 minutes. Remove paper towel and wipe clean. Rinse and dry completely.

Campers an RVs: Easy Laundry Cleaning
No easy access to a laundry machine while you are on the road? Try this novel, but functional, method for washing laundry while camping. Using this solution, a watertight container is used as a "washing machine" to launder clothing while you are driving. The motion of driving works to agitate laundry and clean clothing. You will arrive at your day's destination with clean clothes, ready to rinse fresh and air dry.

1 cup white vinegar
2-3 tablespoons laundry detergent
5 gallons water
watertight container

In watertight container, add white vinegar, water and laundry detergent. Place dirty clothing in container and make certain to seal tightly. Secure in camper and proceed on day's drive. When you arrive at your destination, rinse with clean water and hang outside to dry.

Car: Air Freshener

This is a great solution to make in advance and keep on hand for a quick and easy air freshener in cars. Trial-size spray bottles are perfect for this one!

1/4 cup apple cider vinegar
small, fine mist spray bottle

Fill fine mist spray bottle with undiluted vinegar. Gently mist car interior for a fresh, clean smell anytime.

Car: Ashtrays

white vinegar, undiluted
newspaper or paper towel

Wipe out dirty ashtray with wadded up newspaper or paper towel drenched in white vinegar. Allow to air dry. Vinegar will neutralize away any ashtray odor leaving your car smelling fresh and clean.

Car: Bumper Sticker Removal

white vinegar, undiluted
cloth or small towel

Completely saturate cloth or small towel in vinegar. Do not wring out. Wrap soaked vinegar cloth around bumper where decal is attached. Allow to set undisturbed for 45 minutes. Remove wet towel and pull off sticker. Repeat again, if necessary. You may wish to use soaked towel to further wipe off any residual glue once sticker has been removed.

Car: Chrome

white vinegar, undiluted
clean cloth

Wipe down car chrome with undiluted vinegar. Buff dry to a high shine with a soft, clean cloth.

Car: Chrome Rust Spots

white vinegar, undiluted
aluminum foil
rinse water
wax

Tear off a small piece of aluminum foil and dip it in white vinegar. Rub out small rust spots on chrome until they are completely gone. Rinse away debris and dry completely with a clean towel. Using a small amount of wax, add a thick wax coating to the area that was rusted to protect chrome and prevent new rust spots from forming.

Car: Window Interiors

1/2 cup white vinegar
1/4 cup clean water
paper towels or chamois

Combine white vinegar and water. Use a paper towel or chamois to wipe fingerprints and smudges from interior car windows.

Car: Windshield Washer Cleaner

This is an excellent windshield washer cleaner for a no-streak, no-freeze cleaner.

1/2 cup white vinegar
2 cups rubbing alcohol
1 tablespoon liquid detergent
6 cups water

In a small clean bucket, combine water and liquid detergent. Add vinegar and rubbing alcohol and combine. Pour into windshield washer reservoir.

Car: Vinyl Interiors
1/2 cup white vinegar
1 teaspoon liquid soap
1/2 cup water

Combine all ingredients in a small bowl. Wipe onto vinyl surfaces with a clean cloth. Rinse with clear water and buff dry.

Driveway: Grass Growing in Cracks
white vinegar, undiluted

Pour white vinegar directly into cracks in driveway or sidewalk where grass is growing between the blocks. Check back in a couple of days and repeat, if necessary.

Driveway: Grass Growing in Cracks
2 cups white vinegar
3 tablespoons salt
spray bottle

Combine white vinegar and salt in a spray bottle and swirl to completely dissolve salt (do not place sprayer on bottle until salt has been dissolved). Use this solution to spray onto unwanted grass growing from cracks in driveways or sidewalks.

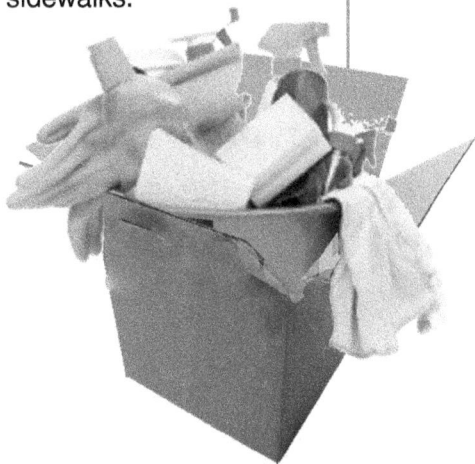

Garage: Brooms

Use this idea to give a second life to an old, about-to-be-discarded broomstick.

1 cup apple cider vinegar
bucket of hot water
knife or scissors

Using a sharp knife or scissors, carefully cut about a third the length of the broom's very worn bristles off, cutting at a deep angle (leaving the short side about 1 inch in length and the longer side about 6 inches in length).

Add vinegar to a bucket of hot water and soak the newly cut broom for about 15 minutes to soften its bristles. Remove broom and shake, getting rid of most of the excess vinegar liquid. Set broom outside in direct sunlight to air dry. When completely dry, use this new angled broom to reach hard to clean floor corners.

Garage: Cement Floor

This simple but powerful solution can help clean a dirty garage floor.

1 cup white vinegar
1 gallon water
shredded newspaper

In a bucket, add white vinegar to a gallon of water. Take a pile of shredded newspaper and pour vinegar solution over it. Toss the wet shredded newspaper over garage floor and sweep with a push broom. Dust and debris will cling to the newspaper, while the white vinegar acts to help neutralize odors.

Garage: Cement Floor

Simple grass clippings will help clean dust and other debris from dirty garage floors.

2 cups apple cider vinegar
grass clippings

Spread handfuls of grass clippings around garage floor. Sprinkle apple cider vinegar over the discarded clippings and allow to set for 10 minutes. Use additional apple cider vinegar if necessary, but it does not need to coat all the clippings entirely. Using a push broom, sweep the cement flooring clean. The resulting garage floor will not only be clean, but the apple cider vinegar also gives the entire garage a fresh smell.

Garage: Cement Floor Oil Stains

This solution is hard working to remove oil stains from a leaky car engine.

1 cup white vinegar
1/2 gallon water
1-2 cups powdered laundry detergent
paper towels

Soak up as much standing oil as possible with paper towels and discard. Sprinkle a heavy coat of powdered laundry detergent over oil stain and allow to absorb. Using a push broom, brush away oil that has now adhered itself to the detergent. Repeat, if necessary until majority of stain is removed.

Add white vinegar to water in a bucket, and pour over the old stained area. Spray away with a garden hose for final rinse.

Garage: Cement Floor Oil Stains
Try this idea to remove hard to clean oil stains on a garage floor.

1 cup white vinegar
1/2 gallon water
2-3 cups unused cat litter
paper towels

Use paper towels to soak up as much oil as possible from garage flooring and discard. Pour a heavy coating of cat litter directly on top of oil stain. Allow it to soak up oil for about 20 minutes. Use a push broom to push away oil-soaked cat litter and discard into a trash can.

Combine white vinegar and water in a bucket and pour over the old stain. Spray with a garden hose to remove any final residue.

Garage: Paintbrushes
1 quart white vinegar

Pour white vinegar into a large, heavy pot and add dirty paintbrushes. Bring to a boil. Cover pot and remove from stovetop and allow to rest for one hour. Place vinegar pot with brushes back on stovetop and bring once again to a gentle boil. Simmer for 20 minutes.

Rinse brushes well, working the softened paint out of the bristles with your fingers or a metal painters comb. For extremely heavy paint encrustations, repeat the process a second time before allowing to air dry.

Garage: Tools
1/4 cup white vinegar
1 quart water

Combine water and white vinegar and use together to wipe away any mineral buildup on metal tools.

Luggage: Odor
1/4 cup white vinegar
clean cloth

Wet cloth with vinegar and wring out excess. Place damp cloth in luggage and close, but do not zipper shut. Allow to set overnight to eliminate odor.

Plastic Picnic Coolers
2 cups white vinegar, divided
1 teaspoon liquid detergent
1 gallon water, plus 1 cup water
extra water for rinsing

Empty a plastic picnic cooler that has become dirty or musty and wipe out all food crumbs and debris. Pour 1 cup white vinegar, liquid detergent and 1 gallon water into cooler. Using a cleaning cloth, make sure solution soaks into all areas of the cooler, including inside the lid. Put lid back onto cooler and allow to set while the outside of the cooler is being cleaned.

To clean the outside of cooler, combine a second cup of vinegar and 1 cup water. Use a cloth to wipe down cooler's exterior. Open cooler and dump out contents. Wipe down the inside and rinse thoroughly. Dry entire cooler.

Window Screens

1 cup white vinegar
1/2 gallon water

Combine white vinegar and water in a bucket, and use sponge to clean dirty window screens. For screens with heavy buildup, pretreat screens prior to sponge cleaning by putting vinegar in a spray bottle and wetting screens first. Allow these screens to set for 10 minutes and then proceed to clean with a wet sponge.

Chapter Eight

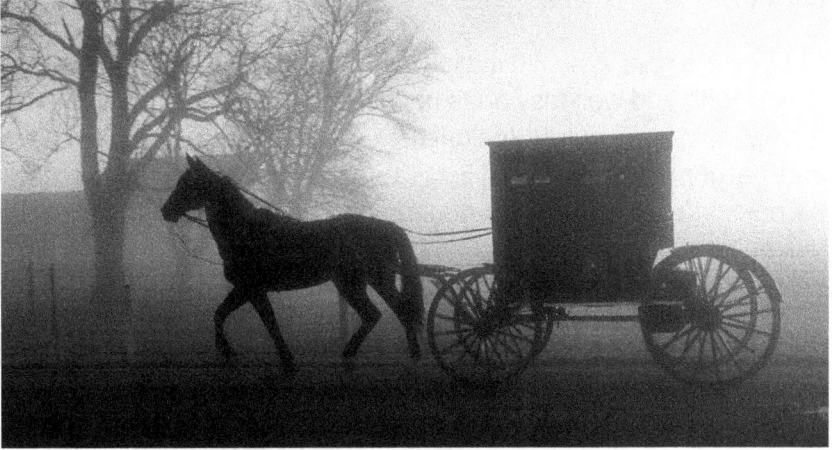

Vinegar & Diet

A recent study from the Center for Disease Control's National Center for Health Statistics shows the obesity rate in the United States now stands at a whopping 39.9%. That is nearly 40% of the U.S. population that is considered obese, and doesn't include people that fall into the "overweight" category. In contrast, rates of Amish obesity are lower, and, depending on the particular Amish sect, can be *sharply l*ower.

So, how is it that some Amish, despite consuming diets which are high in both fat and calories, can exhibit lower rates of obesity than that of the population at large? The majority of their meals consist of foods not only high in carbohydrates, but also refined sugar — two foods the healthcare industry strongly recommends avoiding.

One reason lies in the Amish work ethic. They are renown for their exceptional work drive, laboring long days on their farms, and in local stores and workshops. They are not afraid of hard work, so exercise and physical exertion has become second nature to them. And, with this comes burning off so many of those extra calories consumed at mealtime.

But, it is said in health circles that you cannot out exercise a bad diet. Health and wellness does not necessarily equal input (calories taking in) versus output (calories expended during exercise). One can be underweight, but still not healthy. Likewise, someone can be holding onto a few extra pounds, but be more fit than someone weighing less.

The Problem with "Diets"

As a culture, too often we fall into "diet mode" when we find ourselves overweight. While dieting may shed unwanted pounds in the short term, it is more often than not inadequate in the long term. Soon after completing a diet, pounds begin to creep back on, and we find ourselves right back to where we started, or weighing more than when we began.

The reason this happens is twofold.

First, when we restrict the intake of calories, our bodies naturally go into a self-defense mode and our metabolism is lowered. This means our bodies burn calories more slowly in order to hold onto them as long as possible. It is a natural defense mechanism to avoid starvation. So, calories are not burned at the rate they normally are, which can make weight loss more difficult.

Second, most people, upon completion of a diet, revert to their former eating habits — the very same eating habits that helped cause them to become overweight in the first place (although allowance needs to be made for those people struggling with weight issues due to medical conditions outside of their control).

In both cases, the person dieting winds up in exactly the same position they originally found themselves in, but now feels discouraged and defeated.

Albert Einstein was quoted as saying, "Insanity is doing the same thing over and over, but expecting different results." Simply put, successful weight loss requires a new mindset.

So, how do the Amish stay both healthy and fit, and what role can vinegar play in accomplishing this?

As previously discussed, ongoing wellness and maintaining a healthy weight begins with prevention. The Amish live healthy lives from the get-go, avoiding bad habits such as excessive drinking and drug use to being proactive in adding health-building foods into their daily diet.

One of the very best foods to consider for both healthy living and weight loss is apple cider vinegar. Many people claim to have success in losing unwanted pounds and maintaining a healthy weight through its use. The general thought behind this is that apple cider vinegar, when taken daily with meals:

• Can help kickstart and increase the body's own metabolism

• Burn extra calories through thermogenetics

• Aids the body in digestion

• Increases the feeling of fullness before meals

• Adds essential nutrients to the body that, when depleted, can inhibit proper function of the body, including digestion and the body's ability to properly burn calories

Apple cider vinegar is the vinegar-of-choice for weight loss, due to its particular makeup. Because this type of vinegar is made up of dozens of nutrients and compounds not found in other types of vinegar, it is thought to have a greater potential for weight loss. Many people swear by the simple extra kick their body received from the apple cider vinegar tonic recipes that follow.

In a nutshell, successful weight loss happens most easily when we eat a balanced diet consisting of as many whole, natural foods as possible, exercise regularly (even if it just taking a daily stroll around the neighborhood or working in the flower garden), and seeing if your body reacts by trying an extra boost from apple cider vinegar!

Daily Tonic
2 teaspoons of apple cider vinegar
1 teaspoon of honey
1 glass of water

Combine these three ingredients and consume once a day.

Before Meals
1 teaspoon apple cider vinegar
1 cup of water

To receive the greatest benefit, drink this 10 - 20 minutes before mealtime.

Before Meals #2
1 teaspoon apple cider vinegar
1 teaspoon honey
1 cup water

The addition of honey to this recipe makes it more palatable if the taste of vinegar is too strong. Consume this 10 - 20 minutes before mealtime for the best results.

Index

✂ please cut here

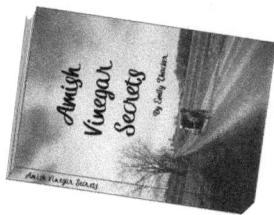

Amish
Vinegar
Secrets

VISA MasterCard DISCOVER AMEX

Exp. date _____

90-DAY MONEY-BACK GUARANTEE

☐ YES! Please rush _____ additional copies of Amish Vinegar Secrets and my FREE copy of the bonus booklet *"Recipes of the Great Depression"* for only $12.95 plus $3.98 postage & handling. I understand that I must be completely satisfied or I can return it within 90 days for a full and prompt refund of my purchase price. The FREE gift is mine to keep regardless. *Want to save even more? Do a favor for a close relative or friend and order two books for only $20 postpaid.*

I am enclosing $_____ by: ☐ Check ☐ Money Order (Make checks payable to James Direct, Inc.)

Charge my credit card Signature _____

Card No. _____

Name _____

Address _____

City _____ State _____ Zip _____

Mail To: JAMES DIRECT, INC. • PO Box 980, Dept. AVS207, Hartville, Ohio 44632
http://www.jamesdirect.com

✂ please cut here

Use this coupon to order "Amish Vinegar Secrets" for a friend or family member -- or copy the ordering information onto a plain piece of paper and mail to:

Amish Vinegar Secrets
Dept. AVS207
PO Box 980
Hartville, Ohio 44632

Preferred Customer Reorder Form

Order this...	If you want a book on...	Cost...	Number of Copies...
Amish Vinegar Secrets	No one knows natural healing and prevention better than the AMISH! This must-read reveals generations worth of all-natural healing remedies and potent cleaning techniques using everyday household vinegar.	$9.95	
The Vinegar Anniversary Book	Completely updated with the latest research and brand new remedies and uses for apple cider vinegar. Handsome coffee table collector's edition you'll be proud to display.	$9.95	
The Magic of Hydrogen Peroxide	An Ounce of Hydrogen Peroxide is worth a Pound of Cure! Hundreds of health cures, household uses & home remedy uses for hydrogen peroxide contained in this breakthrough volume.	$9.95	
The Magic of Baking Soda	*Plain Old Baking Soda A Drugstore in A Box?* Doctors & researchers have discovered baking soda has amazing healing properties! Over 600 health & Household Hints. *Great Recipes Too!*	$9.95	
Amish Gardening Secrets	You too can learn the special gardening secrets the Amish use to produce huge tomato plants and bountiful harvests. Information packed 800-plus collection for you to tinker with and enjoy.	$9.95	
Any combination of the above $9.95 items qualifies for the following discounts...	**Total NUMBER of $9.95 items**		

Order any 2 items for: **$15.95**

Order any 3 items for: **$19.95**

Order any 4 items for: **$24.95**

Order any 5 items for: **$29.95**

Order any 6 items for: **$34.95** and receive 7th item FREE

Any additional items for: **$5 each**

FEATURED SELECTIONS		Total COST of $9.95 items	
The Honey Book	Amazing Honey Remedies to relieve arthritis pain, kill germs, heal infection and much more!	$19.95	
The Cinnamon Book	Research studies have found this amazing spice is loaded with health benefits. Find out how cinnamon can be used in treating common (and not so common) conditions such as diabetes, obesity, arthritis, high cholesterol and a host of other ailments.	$19.95	
Hydrogen Peroxide Formula Guide	FINALLY...No more guesswork! Step-by-step instructions and specific measurements for hundreds of amazing hydrogen peroxide uses. Learn how to use hydrogen peroxide to clean your home, balance pH soil levels, use as a home remedy or beautify your life! It is all here!	$19.95	
Order any 2 or more Featured Selections for only $10 each...	**Postage & Handling**		$3.98*
	TOTAL		

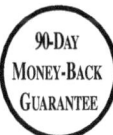

90-DAY MONEY-BACK GUARANTEE

*** Shipping of 10 or more books = $6.96**

Please rush me the items marked above. I understand that I must be completely satisfied or I can return any item within 90 days for a full and prompt refund of my purchase price.

I am enclosing $_____ by: ❏ Check ❏ Money Order (Make checks payable to James Direct Inc)

Charge my credit card Signature _____

Card No. _____ Exp. Date _____

Name _____ Address _____

City _____ State_____ Zip _____

Telephone Number (_____) _____

❏ Yes! I'd like to know about freebies, specials and new products before they are nationally advertised. My email address is: _____

Mail To: **James Direct Inc.** • PO Box 980, Dept. A1432 • Hartville, Ohio 44632
Customer Service (330) 877-0800 • *http://www.jamesdirect.com*

©2018 JDI A267IM

AMISH VINEGAR SECRETS

Learn the Amish way to better health! Studies indicate the Amish have less instances of asthma, cardiovascular disease and some forms of cancer. Learn their secrets to better health using everyday household vinegar to treat common (and not-so-common) illness, prevent sickness before it sets in and have a germ-free household.

THE VINEGAR ANNIVERSARY BOOK

Handsome coffee table edition and brand new information on Mother Nature's Secret Weapon – apple cider vinegar!

THE MAGIC OF HYDROGEN PEROXIDE

Hundreds of health cures & home remedy uses for hydrogen peroxide. You'll be amazed to see how a little hydrogen peroxide mixed with a pinch of this or that from your cupboard can do everything from relieving chronic pain to making age spots go away! Easy household cleaning formulas too!

THE MAGIC OF BAKING SODA

We all know baking soda works like magic around the house. It cleans, deodorizes & works wonders in the kitchen and in the garden. But did you know it's an effective remedy for allergies, bladder infection, heart disorders... *and MORE!*

AMISH GARDENING SECRETS

There's something for everyone in *Amish Gardening Secrets.* This BIG collection contains over 800 gardening hints, suggestions, time savers and tonics that have been passed down over the years in Amish communities and elsewhere.

THE HONEY BOOK

Each page is packed with healing home remedies and ways to use honey to heal wounds, fight tooth decay, treat burns, fight fatigue, restore energy, ease coughs and even make cancer-fighting drugs more effective. Great recipes too!

THE CINNAMON BOOK

Cinnamon is rich in natural healing properties such as being an anti-oxidant, anti-inflammatory, anti-coagulant, anti-microbial, anti-parasitic, anti-tumor – just to name a few! Find out how cinnamon can be used to fight everything from simple cuts and scrapes to chronic health condition, safely and naturally!

HYDROGEN PEROXIDE FORMULA GUIDE

This unique book lists hundreds of home remedy, gardening and cleaning uses for peroxide along with exact measurements and instructions for each use. No mistakes and no guesswork.

* Each Book has its own FREE Bonus!